N. Ichalkaranje, A. Ichalkaranje, L.C. Jain (Eds.)

Intelligent Paradigms for Assistive and Preventive Healthcare

Studies in Computational Intelligence, Volume 19

Editor-in-chief
Prof. Janusz Kacprzyk
Systems Research Institute
Polish Academy of Sciences
ul. Newelska 6
01-447 Warsaw
Poland
E-mail: kacprzyk@ibspan.waw.pl

Further volumes of this series can be found on our homepage: springer.com

Vol. 5. Da Ruan, Guoqing Chen, Etienne E. Kerre, Geert Wets (Eds.)
Intelligent Data Mining, 2005
ISBN 3-540-26256-3

Vol. 6. Tsau Young Lin, Setsuo Ohsuga, Churn-Jung Liau, Xiaohua Hu, Shusaku Tsumoto (Eds.)
Foundations of Data Mining and Knowledge Discovery, 2005
ISBN 3-540-26257-1

Vol. 7. Bruno Apolloni, Ashish Ghosh, Ferda Alpaslan, Lakhmi C. Jain, Srikanta Patnaik (Eds.)
Machine Learning and Robot Perception, 2005
ISBN 3-540-26549-X

Vol. 8. Srikanta Patnaik, Lakhmi C. Jain, Spyros G. Tzafestas, Germano Resconi, Amit Konar (Eds.)
Innovations in Robot Mobility and Control, 2006
ISBN 3-540-26892-8

Vol. 9. Tsau Young Lin, Setsuo Ohsuga, Churn-Jung Liau, Xiaohua Hu (Eds.)
Foundations and Novel Approaches in Data Mining, 2005
ISBN 3-540-28315-3

Vol. 10. Andrzej P. Wierzbicki, Yoshiteru Nakamori
Creative Space, 2005
ISBN 3-540-28458-3

Vol. 11. Antoni Ligęza
Logical Foundations for Rule-Based Systems, 2006
ISBN 3-540-29117-2

Vol. 12. Jonathan Lawry
Modelling and Reasoning with Vague Concepts, 2006
ISBN 0-387-29056-7

Vol. 13. Nadia Nedjah, Ajith Abraham, Luiza de Macedo Mourelle (Eds.)
Genetic Systems Programming, 2006
ISBN 3-540-29849-5

Vol. 14. Spiros Sirmakessis (Ed.)
Adaptive and Personalized Semantic Web, 2006
ISBN 3-540-30605-6

Vol. 15. Lei Zhi Chen, Sing Kiong Nguang, Xiao Dong Chen
Modelling and Optimization of Biotechnological Processes, 2006
ISBN 3-540-30634-X

Vol. 16. Yaochu Jin (Ed.)
Multi-Objective Machine Learning, 2006
ISBN 3-540-30676-5

Vol. 17. Te-Ming Huang, Vojislav Kecman, Ivica Kopriva
Kernel Based Algorithms for Mining Huge Data Sets, 2006
ISBN 3-540-31681-7

Vol. 18. Chang Wook Ahn
Advances in Evolutionary Algorithms, 2006
ISBN 3-540-31758-9

Vol. 19. N. Ichalkaranje, A. Ichalkaranje, L.C. Jain (Eds.)
Intelligent Paradigms for Assistive and Preventive Healthcare, 2006
ISBN 3-540-31762-7

N. Ichalkaranje
A. Ichalkaranje
L.C. Jain
(Eds.)

Intelligent Paradigms for Assistive and Preventive Healthcare

Springer

N. Ichalkaranje
University of South Australia
Adelaide
Australia

L.C. Jain
University of South Australia
Adelaide
Australia

A. Ichalkaranje
Independent Living Centre
Adelaide
Australia

Library of Congress Control Number: 2006920196

ISSN print edition: 1860-949X
ISSN electronic edition: 1860-9503
ISBN-10 3-540-31762-7 Springer Berlin Heidelberg New York
ISBN-13 978-3-540-31762-3 Springer Berlin Heidelberg New York

Springer is a part of Springer Science+Business Media
springer.com

Printed in The Netherlands

Typesetting: by the author and techbooks using a Springer LaTeX macro package

Printed on acid-free paper SPIN: 11418337 89/techbooks 5 4 3 2 1 0

This book is dedicated to our students.

Foreword

Intelligent systems have had a tremendous impact in various fields including business, science, technology and healthcare. This impact is largely due to readily and widely available computing power.

Many researchers all over the world are using intelligent techniques in assistive and preventive healthcare. Assistive technology will have a major impact not only in supporting independent living but also in supporting functional abilities of all people in need of support. Devices like intelligent wheel chairs, walking aids, hearing aids, reading aids, context-aware computing and smart homes are not dreams of the future but a reality today. Their improvement and wide-spread acceptance by those who need such devices will continue to increase.

This book presents top-notch contributions on assistive and preventive healthcare by active and well-known researchers in the field. The areas covered are not meant to be exhaustive but enough to create wide-spread interest among the community in the applications of intelligent paradigms in assistive and preventive healthcare.

I wish to congratulate whole-heartedly the contributors for their vision and their concern for the community we live in.

Professor Dr Hermann Maurer,
Dean, Faculty of Computer Science,
Graz University of Technology,
Graz
Austria

Preface

This book presents some of the recent advances in assistive and preventive healthcare in intelligent environment. As the world is becoming increasingly aware of the needs of people with disabilities, researchers are finding new technologies and applications to assist disabled people in performing the everyday activities which able-bodied people often take for granted.

Chapter 1 describes remote healthcare for patients in remote areas and in areas that have few health professionals. In this age of decreasing resources, there are many benefits associated with remote healthcare. It allows a greater range of expertise for patients (eg. with teleconferencing). With technology becoming more affordable, these applications have the potential to become available at all healthcare facilities and to all patients. Smaller devices to monitor health will allow enhanced monitoring. Wireless monitoring devices will allow patients to be monitored in their own environments performing their usual activities, therefore giving a more accurate diagnosis of their health. The author introduces the 'wireless sensor network' and 'an evolvable network of tiny sensors' (ANTS). The author also discusses technologies that are useful for remote healthcare.

Chapter 2 describes multimedia applications for health professionals. An example of this is in record keeping, thereby minimising the time spent on this tedious but necessary task and allowing more time for patient contact. Other areas where multimedia applications are useful include establishing a diagnosis (eg. using inference rules), and remote access to information. The author works with her team at the University of Veszprem. Examples of technology developed by the author's team include programs for children with limited vision or hearing, for motor-impaired children, for stroke patients, and for aphasic patients.

Chapter 3 gives a comprehensive summary of the uses of virtual reality. For example, virtual reality has uses in teaching and training of staff (eg. for complex techniques or concepts). Virtual reality is an inexpensive teaching modality which eliminates the risk to patients, and allows for more efficient education. There are also uses in diagnosis, simulation of surgery (eg. during planning), and networking. It can be used in patient rehabilitation, for example, after brain injury (eg. virtual reality to simulate everyday tasks). There are also uses outside healthcare, for example, teaching children to cross a street. The authors go on to describe the virtual reality programs which they have developed.

Chapter 4 presents digital talking books, which are a multimedia version of a print publication. Digital talking books enable access to information for those who are unable to access printed information. The chapter highlights the 'DAISY Consortium', a non-profit organisation founded to facilitate the transition from analogue to digital talking books, with special attention given to integration with mainstream technology to allow access to information for people with print disabilities.

Chapter 5 provides a review of existing devices to assist with locomotion for people with visual impairments. There is an analysis of the shortcomings of existing systems (eg. infrared sensors, ultrasonic sensors, and laser telemeters). People with visual impairments have limited autonomy in complex, changing environments (eg. shopping malls). They need to rely largely on memory, and if they are fortunate, guide dogs. Electronic devices can provide advance warnings for these people, therefore allowing anticipation, and greater independence. The authors also discuss new systems (eg. Personal Digital Assistants).

Chapter 6 presents a multimedia system called MIMIZU for people with visual impairments. This system uses a refreshable tactile display and a stylus pen. The system allows blind users to communicate tactile image information with each other.

Chapter 7 presents the use of information and communications technology for people with hearing impairments. This chapter explores the use of various applications of this technology, for example, sign language videos to allow effective communication for people with a hearing impairment.

Chapter 8 presents a gait training system which uses a sling and force plates on a round track. The aim of the device is to supplement or enhance training by a therapist, rather than replace the therapist. The device allows the treatment of multiple patients simultaneously. The device decreases the load on therapists, resulting in many advantages (eg. increased safety and efficiency) for therapists and patients. Future potential enhancements for this system are also discussed.

This book is a valuable addition to the growing field of assistive technology. It provides insight as well as direction for those interested in the technology aspect as well as those interested in the healthcare aspects. We commend the authors on their foresight in the area of assistive technology. We also acknowledge the expertise and time of the reviewers. We appreciate the assistance of Berend Jan van der Zwaag during the final preparation of manuscript. Finally, we also wish to thank Springer-Verlag for their support.

Australia
07 January 2006

A. Ichalkaranje
N.Ichalkaranje
L.C. Jain

Table of Contents

1. Ubiquitous Healthcare: Technology and Service

Yung Bok Kim[1], Sun K. Yoo[2] and Daeyoung Kim[3]

[1]Department of Computer Engineering,
Sejong University, Seoul, Korea
yungbkim@sejong.ac.kr
[2]Department of Medical Engineering,
Center for Emergency Medical Informatics,
Yonsei University College of Medicine, Seoul, Korea
sunkyoo@yumc.yonsei.ac.kr
[3]Information and Communications University (ICU),
119 Munji-Dong, Yuseong-Gu, 305-714, Daejon, Korea
kimd@icu.ac.kr

Abstract. Ubiquitous healthcare is introduced in terms of technology and service, considering the current technology as well as the future technology and services. In the first section, we introduce the key techniques of ubiquitous healthcare for next-generation medical treatment services. In the second section, we introduce the wireless sensor network (WSN) and ANTS (an Evolvable Network of Tiny Sensors). In the last section, we discuss real-time health-monitoring network for the disabled and elderly people using an inexpensive and effective Web server and health-monitoring sensors in a wrist phone.

1 Key Techniques of Ubiquitous Healthcare

1.1 Introduction

The development of high speed Internet technology and by the use of a wireless network enable medical multimedia systems to support numerous data types (video, audio and biological data). This in turn, made it possible to effectively provide medical treatments to the patients remotely and to help prevent disease [1] [2]. Ubiquitous healthcare system can be regarded as the combination of the Internet and biological measuring devices to manage patients' disease without the limitation of time and space and without resorting to specific types of measuring device. In short, it is an upgraded version of the biological measuring devices with data transmission capability. There is a tendency for the measuring devices to be smaller, able to be attached using wireless, digitized and using less power [3]. The user may util-

Y.B. Kim et al.: *Ubiquitous Healthcare: Technology and Service*, Studies in Computational Intelligence (SCI) **19**, 1–35 (2006)
www.springerlink.com

ize this to monitor health condition and predict potential hazardous conditions irrespective of the time and place. This section introduces the core technologies for a medical multimedia system. The portable medical devices being researched for each phase of the ubiquitous healthcare system and some of the basic requirements for an effective ubiquitous healthcare system are considered.

1.2 Design Consideration for Medical Multimedia System

The functions of a medical multimedia system are the support of tele-consultation for timely decision-making with regard to patient transfer, accurate instructions for the treatment of the patient, and to help of remote medical specialists. In order to describe precisely the status of a patient to a remote medical specialist, the system includes multimedia components: ECG (Electrocardiogram), BP (Blood Pressure), respiration, oxygen saturation (SpO_2), temperature, systolic and diastolic pressures, heart rate, radiological images, patient records, full-quality video and video conferencing [4]. Table 1 shows the specified design constraints for those multimedia components [5].

Table 1 Design Constraints for Medical Multimedia System

Data type	Priority	Real-time	Remarks
ECG wave	High	Yes	12 bits resolution, 300 Hz sampling ratio
Respiration, BP, and SpO_2 wave	High	Yes	12 bits resolution, 200 Hz sampling ratio
SpO_2 value, systolic pressure, diastolic pressure, temperature, heart rate	High	Yes	Update once per 30 seconds
Radiological images (X-ray, CT, MR etc.)	Low	No	Capture by either DICOM 3.0 or a digital camera interface
Medical record	Low	No	Capture by digital camera
Full-quality video	Medium	Yes	640 X 480 resolution, 30 frames/second
Audio in video conferencing	High	Yes	Must not disturb conversation
Video in video conferencing	Low	Yes	320 X 240 resolution

The multimedia application software performs the control, manipulation and compression /decompression required for transmitting and receiving multimedia over the network. As shown in Fig. 1, the application software is defined by a set of objects organized in different layers, which enables the easy and unified inte-gration of the system with modular blocks. The lowest layer consists of the data acquisition drivers, a TCP/IP socket for network protocol and a kernel for the user interface.

The middle layer, between the lowest and highest layers (application software), consists of the managing software, filters and dedicated blocks.

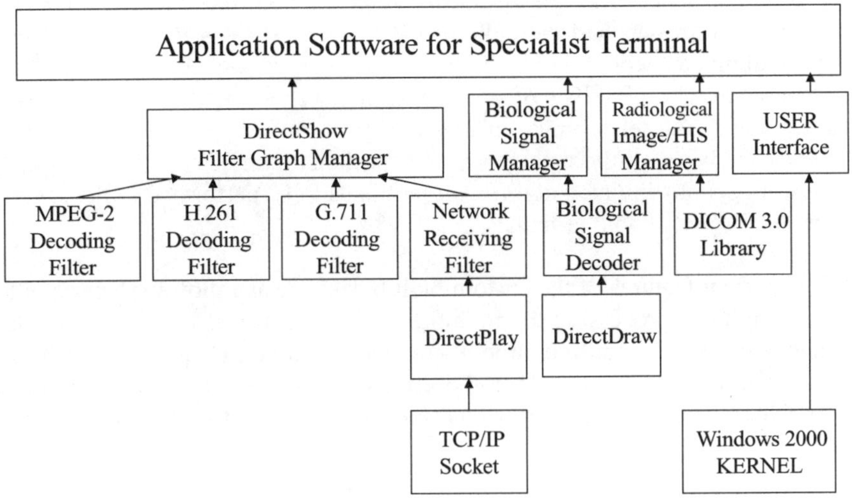

Fig. 1. Software Configuration for Specialist Terminal

- The custom-built blocks in the middle layer are written in visual C++ as a COM (Component Object Model), are based on DirectShow, DirectPlay and DirectDraw (all Microsoft Co.). The DirectShow filter graph manager handles most of the functions needed for the multimedia streams, including MPEG-2 encoding/decoding, H.320 encoding/decoding and the transmitting/receiving of the multimedia streams over the network. DirectShow has a multimedia architecture that enables the application to have very detailed control over the media streams, and uses a "filter" paradigm as a component for composing filter graphs. DirectPlay, under DirectShow filters, handles the transmission and reception of the multimedia streams over the TCP/IP (Transmission Control Protocol/Internet Protocol), while DirectDraw opens the application path for the management of the add-on graphics controller for a fast display. The application software collects multimedia streams and passes them to the appropriate blocks.
- The custom-built encoding filters (H.261 and G.711) compress the low-quality video and audio in real-time, to activate the videoconference.
- The custom-built biological signal manager collects biological signals from the patient monitor, and passes them to both the custom-built biological encoder and to DirectDraw. These compress and display the biological signals, in real-time, respectively.
- The custom-built radiological image/HIS (Hospital Information System) man-

ager initiates the off-line DICOM protocol, in order to retrieve radiological images from the PACS archive. It interprets the content of DICOM files, in order to identify individual image frames, using a custom-built DICOM 3.0 library. In addition, it performs the JPEG decoding for both the DICOM compatible compressed images, and the radiological image/medical record files, produced by the digital camera.

- The user interface consists of simple menus for choosing the functions and the tele-pointer. The tele-pointer enables the synchronous operation on the shared workspace between the emergency and specialist terminals, and is designed to allow all actions initiated at different terminals to be performed in the same order and fashion at both terminals.

The important features of the custom-built blocks are as follows: Their computational capability in processing the multimedia streams in real-time. Their modular structures allowing the configuration of internal functions. Their unified controllability for top-level applications for the effective management of the multimedia streams which depend on the individual media priority and buffer assignment requests.

1.3. Design Considerations for Portable U-healthcare

The service process of the U-healthcare system using portable devices as illustrated in Fig. 2 is as follows: Measurement of Biological Signal/ Analysis. The Display of Signal/ Data transfer and the recording and diagnosis of transferred data. Looking at each phase of the four-step process. The measurement phase requires a composite function, network, non-expensive, light, unconfined and continuous measurement in order to acquire a great deal of various health indices. The monitoring process requires module information from PDA (Portable Digital Assistant), laptop PC, cellular phone and other devices. The measured data shall be analyzed and transferred to applicable medical organization. When the data is transferred through a wireless network environment, it shall have an interface with hospitals and/or other medical organization in order to prove the reliability of the analyzed data.

The sensor that saves the data requires a secure, private, back-up capable system and recoverable function. To implement this type of system, the following four major elements must be taken into account.

- Small and low powered device for mobility purpose
- Elimination of motion artifact in the received signal to ensure the integrity of information
- Data compression to fit the fixed bandwidth available
- Data transfer in a wireless environment

1.3.1 Necessity for a Small and Low Powered Device

In order to minimize the size of the device design with low power, the analog circuitry must be reformatted as much as possible as digital circuitry and controlled by the program.

In general, the analog circuitry is used as signal amplifier and filters to eliminate so and 60Hz noise due to the power line and also any ambient signal created by ambient light. Regarding to the elimination of ambient light, band rejection filter is normally used for ECG and de-multiplexing technique by means of multi-wavelength for SpO_2.

The analog circuit blocks can be replaced by the digital processing programs using the minimum analog circuitry for amplification and the anti-aliasing filter. That is, the conversion of the analog circuitry into the digital circuitry permits a small measuring device and minimizes the distortion caused by the non-linear characteristics of amplitude and the phase inherent in analog circuitry.

1.3.2 Elimination of Motion Artifact in Signal

Removing the motion artifact from measured biological signals is one of the important issues to be tackled for accurate measurement, and is particularly relevant when the human is in motion. The motion artifact, caused by changes in optical probe coupling, patient anatomy, optical properties of tissue, and the complex combinations of all these effects, causes a considerable deterioration in the shape of measured biological signals. The motion artifact is similar to the biological and they mostly occupy the same frequency band. Hence, the elimination of the motion artifact is an essential step in ubiquitous healthcare as the system requires a continuous measurement of the daily physiological parameter when the person is moving about in everyday life.

The following three approaches are commonly used to eliminate the motion artifact. The first method is to record a reference signal from a standstill patient. By comparing the measured signal with the reference signal, the patient movement component is identified. The motion artifact contaminated interval is then replaced by the previously recorded signal. This error concealment method requires an accurate measurement of which contains the reference signal and accurate determination of deformed signal which contains the patient's movement. The second method, especially for the SpO_2, is to use a ring type measuring device to maximize the contact between skin and the ring. This arrangement also minimizes the external impact on the sensor by minimizing the gap between the ring and skin. This method meets the elimination of the motion artifact as well as portability requirements. The third method utilizes Independent Component Analysis (ICA).

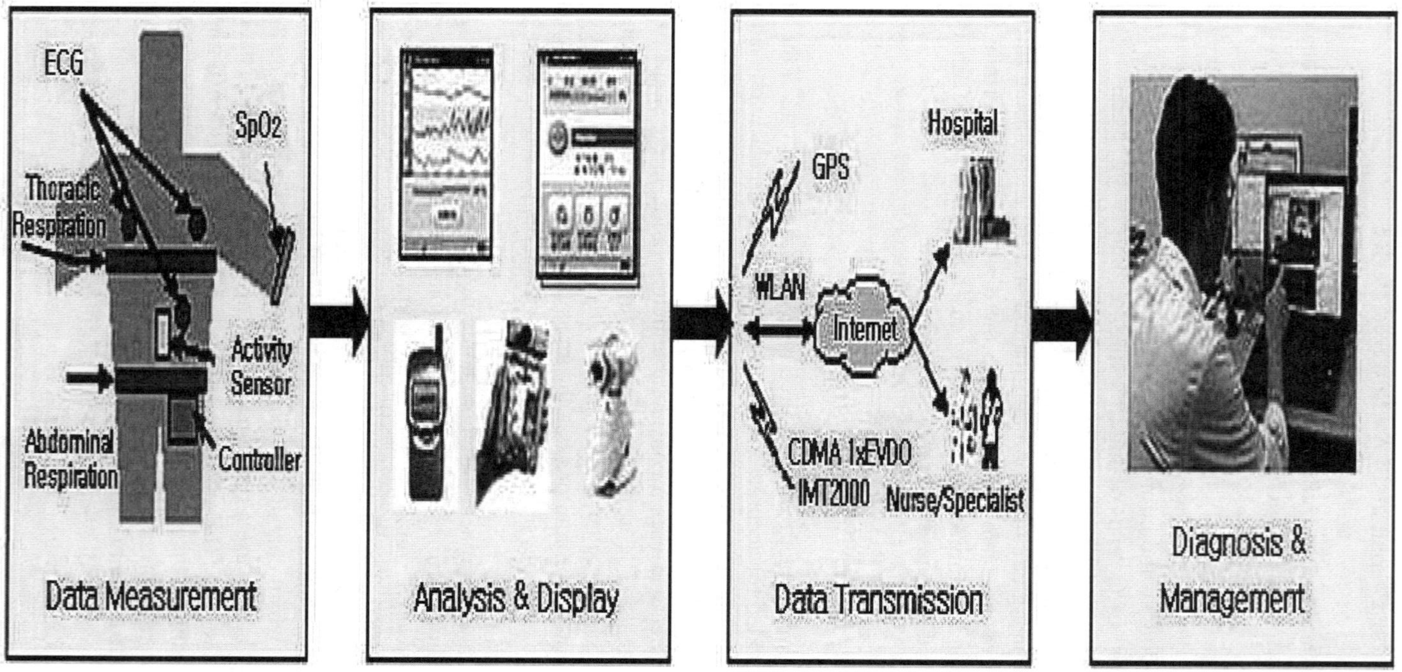

Fig. 2. Service Process of U-healthcare System using Portable Device

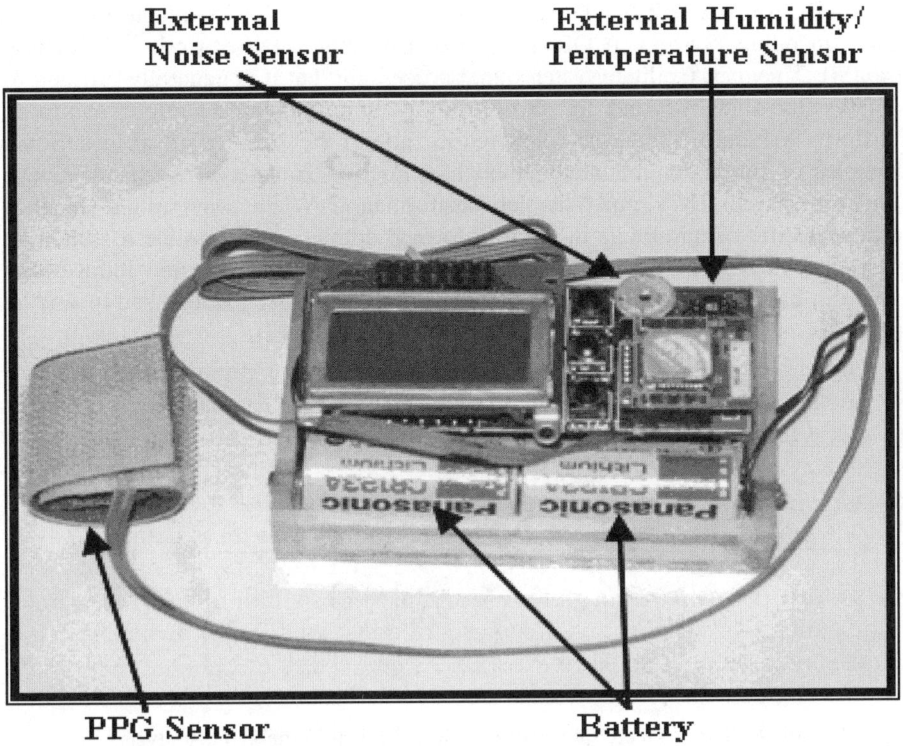

Fig. 3. The Portable Bio-signal Measurement Device.

The underlying assumption in this method is that physiological signal and the motion artifact are independent of each other. For example, Electrocardiography (ECG) or SpO_2 are signals produced by heart beat, whereas the motion artifact signals are attributed by physical movement. ICA can recover original source signals from observed mixtures of unknown signals, emitted by physical objects or sources. Among many applications researched for many years, one of challenging ICA applications is to separate weak signals from multiple sources contaminated with artifacts and noise, which is particularly suitable for bio-signal enhancement [6]. ICA has been successfully applied to bio-signal enhancement in signals contaminated by the motion artifact.

1.3.3 Data Compression

To transfer patient's biological signals via wireless Internet or cellular phone, it is necessary to compress the data size while preserving clinically important biological signal shape for proper diagnosis. For a number of years in the past, many studies were conducted in either the time domain or the transform domain. In time domain method, signals are directly handled in time domain typical methods are: Turning

Point (TP), Amplitude Zone Time Epoch Coding (AZTEC), Coordinate Reduction Time Encoding System (CORTES), and Difference Pulse Code Modulation (DPCM). They can facilitate faster signal processing, but it is generally difficult to compress the signal beyond 3:1. In order to attain an increased compression ratio, transform domain methods are employed in spite of the existing signal loss. Some examples of transform domain method are: Fourier Transform, Karhunen-Loeve Transform (KLT), DCT, and Wavelet transformation. When converting a signal to be in a specific certain range in the transformed domain, it is possible to obtain an energy packing property which is necessary for a high compression ratio. Many transform-based bio-signal compression algorithms have been researched to find an optimized use of storage capacity and network bandwidth [7].

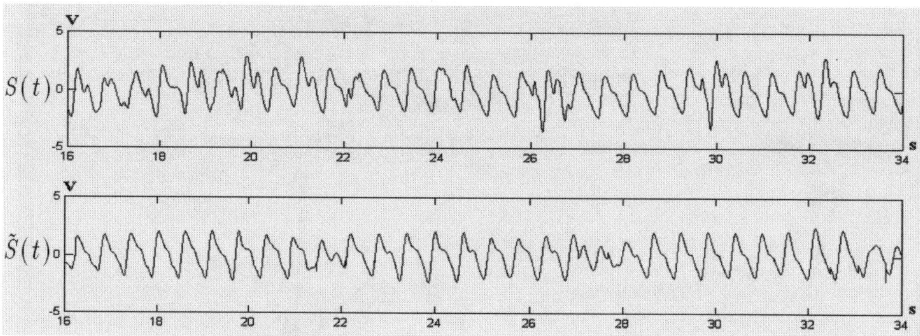

Fig. 4. Motion Artifact reduced SpO_2 Signal by Independent Component Analysis

Among these methods wavelet transform based algorithms have received a great deal of attention. This is because of their easy implementation and efficiency due to their good localization property in the time and frequency domains.

Fig. 4 shows compressed ECG signal using a 6-layer wavelet transformation. After wavelet transformation, the transformed data starts to align in order from the lowest frequency band to highest frequency bands. The lowest frequency band has most of the energy concentrated. It is then possible to increase the compression ratio. In addition, the recursive threshold could be applied to each band in order to compose partitioned wavelet conversion tree. Different bands split according to wavelet transformation enables a gradual transmission having different qualities (progressive transmission). Fig. 5 shows three ECG signals for different compression ratios.

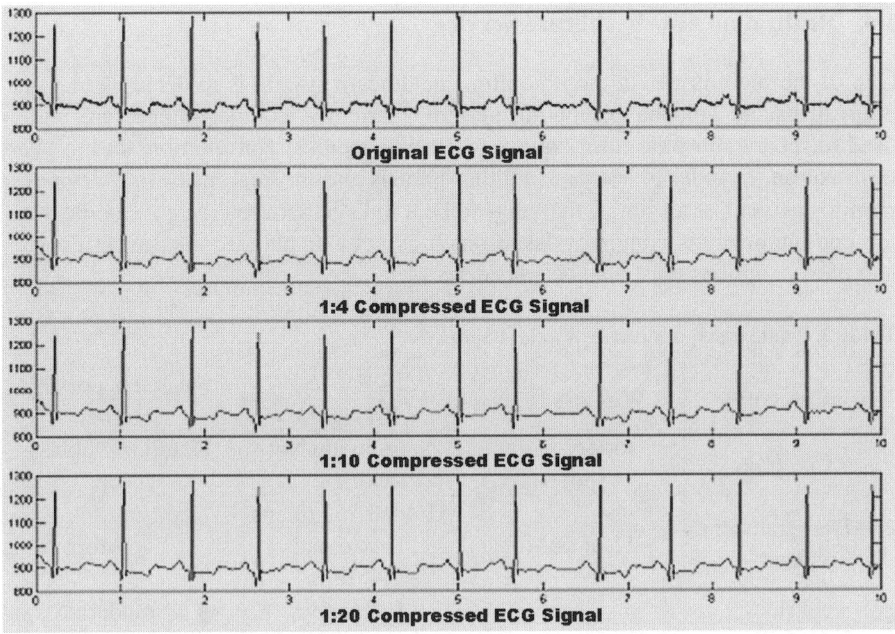

Fig. 5. ECG Signal Compression by means of Wavelet Transformation with different Compression Ratios.

1.3.4 Data Transfer in a Wireless Environment

When transmitting the acquired data to a medical organization in a wireless environment, it is possible that a burst of a random error might occur in the communication channel. These errors will have an adverse impact in the received data. To protect the data from these errors, FEC (Forward Error Correction) and ARQ (Automatic Repeat Request) methods are widely used. FEC transmits error-correcting codes with the original code and ARQ retransmits data upon the receiver's request. FEC does not require retransmission of signal, and it can be done in a short time. It is mostly used in emergency situations, and the ARQ method is used in non-emergency situations. In spite of the long processing time, ARQ accurately sends the information to the medical organization. This step is also related to transmission protocol. The transport layer uses this step to determine whether to use TCP or UDP. In a wireless environment, UDP is more frequently used than TCP. Although TCP guarantees stable data transmission, in wireless environment it might lead to a significant delay in data transmission due to continuous error. In real-time transmission, RTP (Real Time Protocol) and RTCP (Real Time Control Protocol) are also used on top of UDP so as to ensure the transmission reliability and QoS (Quality of Service).

1.4. Realization of U-healthcare Service

One of the main issues in the ubiquitous healthcare system is to decide which medium to use to link the computing system. Currently, cellular phones are widely used to receive hospital information, to reserve medical consultation, and to share information. In order to combine cellular phones and medical measuring devices to monitor patients at all times, there has to be a linkage between the environment and the communications company. Issues such as cellular phones, measuring devices, and power supplies must also be considered.

Table 2. Comparison of diverse Wireless Services

Category	Wireless LAN	1x EV-DO IMT2000	2.3GHz portable Internet
Coverage	Indoor / Hot spot	Nationwide Network	Outdoor, Public Facilities
Data transfer speed	~11 or 54Mbps	Upload 153.6kbps Download ~2.4Mbps	~3Mbps
Price	Cheap	Expensive	moderate
Mobility	Within 5km/h	Beyond 100km/h	~60km/h
Device	Desktop, Laptop	Cell Phone, PDA	Laptop, PDA
Members (per base station)	Tens	Hundreds	Hundreds
Service type	Hi-speed internet	Mobile Telecom	Hi-speed Internet

As seen in Table 2, wireless LAN has a capability of at least 11Mbps transmission speed. Bluetooth enables the communication between measuring devices. CDMA 1X EV-DO, is capable of high speed mobility, but is expensive and has low data transfer speed. Lastly, portable Internet provides a 60km/h mobility and has a high speed data transfer capability. The portable provides an acceptable solution for all the main issues: portability, communications, and power. In the future, when IPv6 will be commonly used, all measuring devices shall have specified IP addresses, and this will facilitate individual remote control and identification.

The final version of the healthcare service shall be as depicted in Fig. 6. A biological measuring device will be attached to patient's body. The monitoring process will be conducted at regular intervals. When unusual signal is detected it will be transmitted to the appropriate medical service center using either wireless or satellite means. The medical center shall maintain the patient's information using the customer database. The doctor in charge of specialized medical agency shall provide the diagnosis and any required prescription. In case of critical situations,

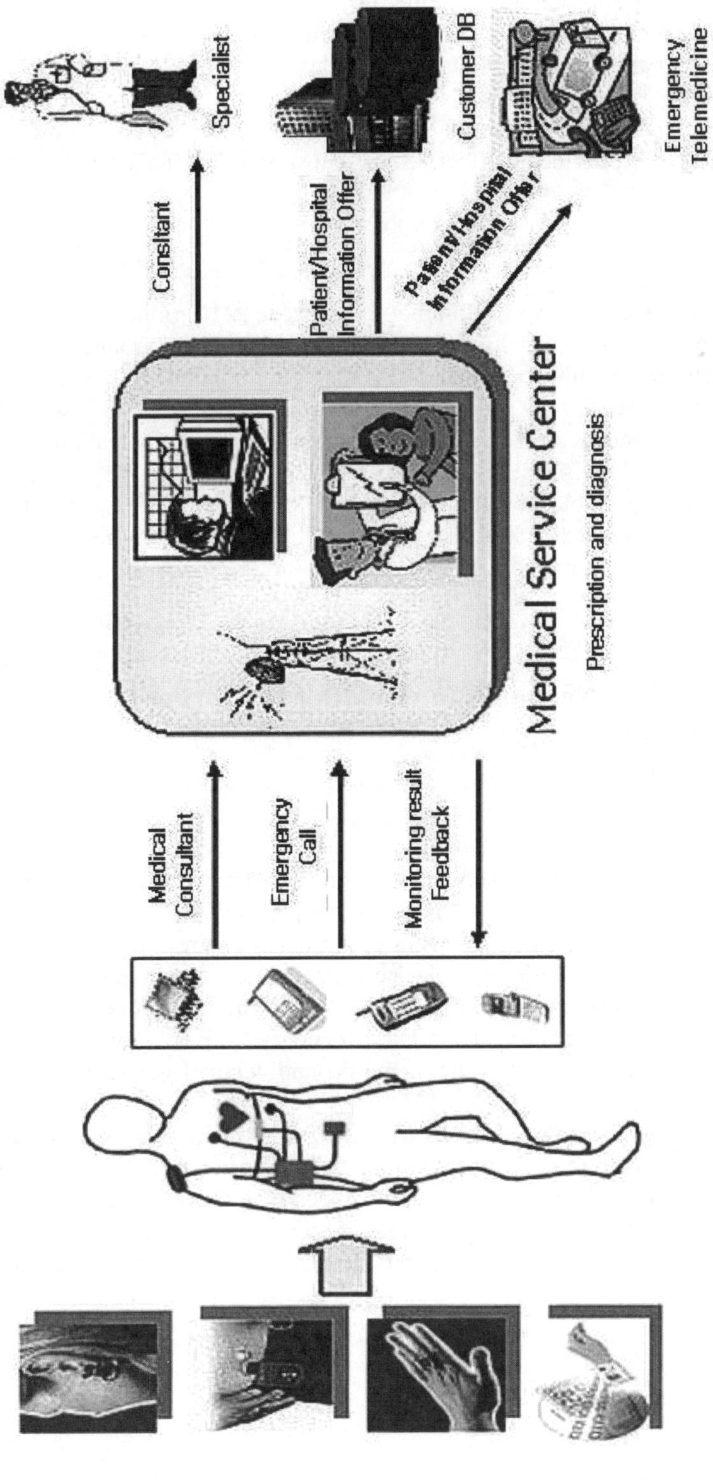

Fig. 6. Overview of Ubiquitous Healthcare Service

the doctor shall take appropriate measures to have the emergency device call an emergency medical center providing urgent first aid.

The healthcare patient shall be able to check his or her health information anywhere at any time without constraint. The medical agency in charge, on the other hand, shall observe the patient's health condition at all times and take the most suitable medical action to provide an effective medical support for the patient.

1.5 Future Prospect

To date, the number of high speed Internet users exceeds 10 million and the computing system is being introduced in Korea. This advanced IT environment makes it possible to satisfy the healthcare demands. As the aging population increases, ubiquitous healthcare service is now proposed as a medical service.

Most ubiquitous healthcare services utilize mobile telecommunications to provide medical consultation, but it is only in the introduction stage. We are all aware that many different portable devices will be developed and the data transferable bandwidth will be expanded and mobility improved. The ubiquitous healthcare user shall receive high quality medical services and prompt treatment in an emergency situation.

2 Wireless Sensor Networks for Health Monitoring and Medical Care

2.1 Introduction

The exciting new field of sensor networks is attracting much attention and is considered to be one of the most interesting research topics today. The work started by visionaries several years ago, now provides prospects of future users. Today's sensor nodes powered with batteries or solar cells provide bi-directional communication to other devices forming networks for data gathering and processing. Sensor devices may be greatly miniaturized and harvest energy from the environment, it is likely they will communicate with other networks and devices integrated in our environments.

The potential of such wireless sensor networks (WSN) is driving government and industries to make important investments in the field. The burst of the sensor device production will provide the basis for a shared experience for all. There are several challenges yet to overcome. The development of software infrastructure has important challenges to overcome in order to make the Sensor Networks part of our every day life.

The range of applications derived from the present efforts in the field of WSN is wide. The first attempts to bring experimental WSN out of the laboratory, now has been used for habitat monitoring [8][9] and also for some similar indoor experiments involving environment control and actuation [10]. Various applications are developed including some social researches focused in human interaction [11]. Several architectures and Operating Systems have arisen and TinyOS [12] is the most popular one.

Recently, a new application for health monitoring and medical care for WSN is gaining popularity amongst researchers and it gives good promises for future practical uses. In this chapter, we will introduce this new field of work and the most active research in the area. We will also introduce ANTS: this is an Evolving Network of Tiny Sensors. ANTS is a new architecture for the development of sensor networks which we hope will help to overcome challenges in exciting field. We will describe some of our research in ANTS to show how it will contribute to the field of WSN in general and medical care in particular.

The rest of the chapter is organized as follows: Section 2.2 discusses applications of WSN in the field of health monitoring and medical care. It provides an introduction and a summary of important ongoing research. In section 2.3, we show the ANTS architecture and discuss several of its functionalities together with applications. Finally section 2.4 gives a summary of the introduced material.

2.2 Health Monitoring and Medical Care Applications using WSN

The need for health monitoring is increasing and its application is becoming feasible with wireless sensor network technology. By adopting tiny wireless sensor devices with a specific health monitoring system, regular patients and elderly people can be observed irrespective of time and place. Vital sign sensors are attached to the patient, allowing continuous monitoring of the physical status. These health monitoring systems are not totally new. However, health monitoring with wireless sensor networks has some outstanding features comparing with traditional medical healthcare systems.

In the past, a number of wireless medical monitors were introduced. Popular health monitor products are Electrocardiographs (EKGs), pulse oximeters, blood pressure monitors, heart rate and maternal uterine monitors. They made use of frequency bands for blue-tooth, analog Wireless Medical Telemetry Service (WMTS), or IEEE 802.11 wireless LAN, for their communication system. This technology was large and communication was limited to fixed terminals. The patient was forced to carry heavy devices. Alternatively, the systems needed to be located next to the immobile patient beds. Such monitoring systems were generally cumbersome and could restrict patients' movements. Monitored data has seldom traditionally been delivered to healthcare systems via a network to provide an integrated result.

A wireless sensor network based health monitoring provides a totally different healthcare system scenario. Sensor nodes are small and generally use battery rather than power cables. In spite of their size, they can communicate with other sensor nodes, and consequently data from attached sensors is easily transferred to the health monitoring system. This freedom prevents patients from feeling they are under observation, and monitoring of various body status can be sensed and checked in a real-time manner without any notification or administrative managements. Should the monitored patient go to a sudden emergency state, programmed sensor network actuators might automatically make emergency calls and the monitoring system would start sending video images along with sensed vital sign data to relevant medical personnel. If required, sensor node networks could become large enough to cover complete hospital complexes or home areas having thousands of sensor nodes.

A sensor network's general features such as tiny sensor nodes, network construction and self-configuration make its possible use in a medical care monitoring application. However sensor network technology itself is still far from the requirements of a medical care system. This is because initially it is not intended to be used for health-monitoring applications. We present a list of requirements for a health-care monitoring sensor network:

- *Reliable data communication*: Most importantly, data communication should be reliable enough to send patient vital signs in real-time. Due to the wireless' system characteristics and the limited capability of the sensor nodes, a reliable communication system must be considerably improved.
- *Wearable sensor nodes*: When the health sensors are integrated into a hardware node, the size should be small enough for comfortable wear.
- *System Security*: Sensed data reveals personal information such as health information, habit and movements. For security reliable systems are necessary.
- *Sensor nodes mobility*: As a result of the patients mobility the topology will continually change. Measures to cope with this must be evolved.

CodeBlue [13] is a one of the most famous health monitoring systems using wireless sensor networks. CodeBlue integrates sensor nodes and other wireless devices into a disaster response setting to provide medical care monitoring. The features include ad-hoc network formation, resource naming and discovery, security and in-network aggregation of sensor-produced data. This development includes a range of medical sensors integrated with the commonly-used Mica2, MicaZ and Telos remote design. Fig. 7 shows CodeBlue sensor node design.

CodeBlue infrastructure in Fig. 8 addresses the discovery and naming mechanism in its communication pathway and its robust routing to connect other sensor nodes. To ensure quality of service, CodeBlue adopts prioritization of critical data so that important data such as vital sign always take precedence over other traffic. In addition, CodeBlue supports the security mechanism and location tracking. Fig. 8 shows the CodeBlue infrastructure.

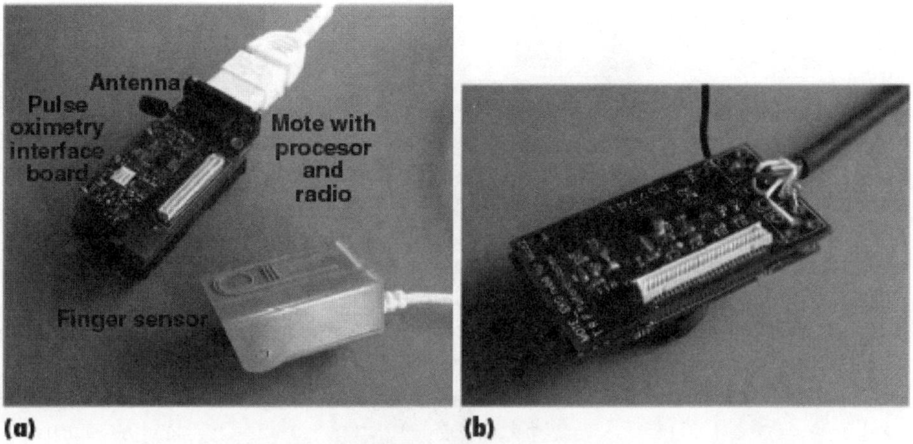

Fig. 7. CodeBlue (a) Pulse Oximeter (b) two-lead Electrocardiogram

Another related research project is the wireless body area network for health monitoring developed by Jovanov *et al.* [14]. Their work aims to support ubiquitous affordable healthcare. The main architecture consists of a three-tier monitoring system. The components are a wireless body area network (WBAN), personal server and healthcare providing server. An example of the architecture is shown in Fig. 9

2.3 ANTS Platform for Healthcare Applications

The ANTS, an Evolving Network of Tiny Sensors, constitutes our particular WSN design to address the challenges imposed by a dynamic future. Contrary to other architectures which rely on static behaviors, ANTS is built with the idea of providing adaptability for a dynamically changing environment, particularly coupling with the needs of the inherently dynamic healthcare monitoring systems. Moreover, advanced features of ANTS such as localization can provide important services in medical care environments.

As depicted in Fig. 10, ANTS architecture includes all the necessary modules to provide a complete and effective system. The ANTS has all in its own hardware design [15] to provide the latest technological trends, together with a new Operating System [16] with powerful new features. The ANTS network architecture and communication protocols [17] deals with the challenges of information transmission and advanced features such as mobility and localization. ANTS synchronization, security and power management contain the foundation of our work, serving as the base for several middleware and application layer designs such as context awareness or a UPnP based management system [18].

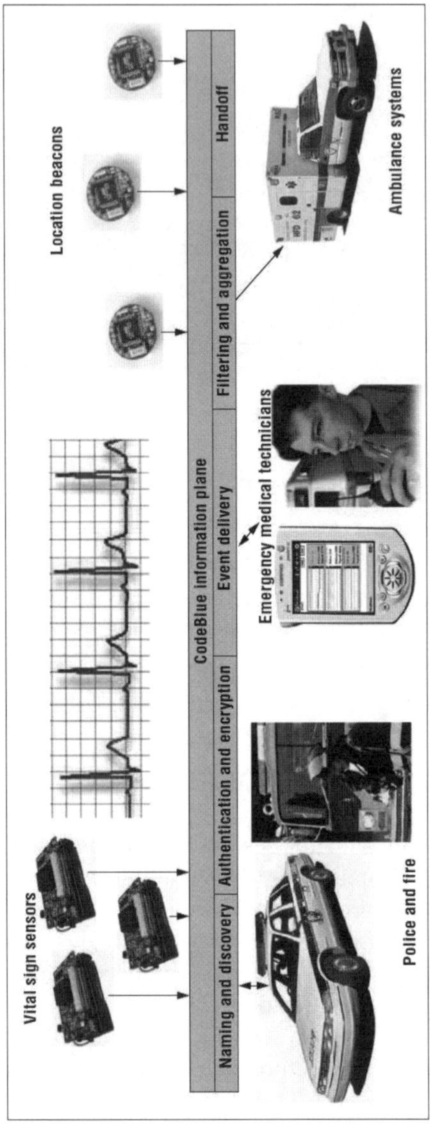

Fig. 8. CodeBlue Infrastructure

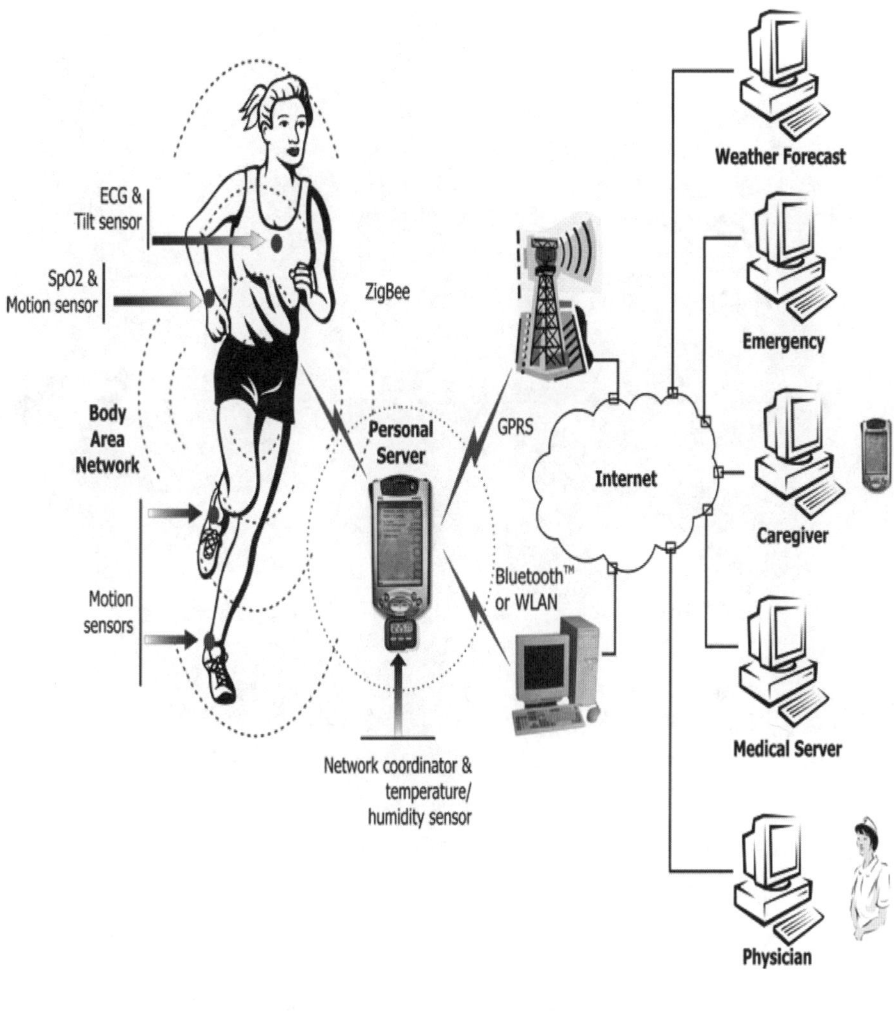

Fig. 9. Wireless Body Area Network of Intelligent Sensors for Patient Monitoring

The ANTS research team has been recently involved in several medical care research projects, such as the E-Health Project developed at the Information and Communications University, South Korea. The project developed a Grid-based PUG (Physio-Ubiquitous Grid) system to analyze and process data obtained from ECG (Electrocardiogram) equipment. The system was designed to include wireless sensor networks in the home environment to collect ECG data from the patient.

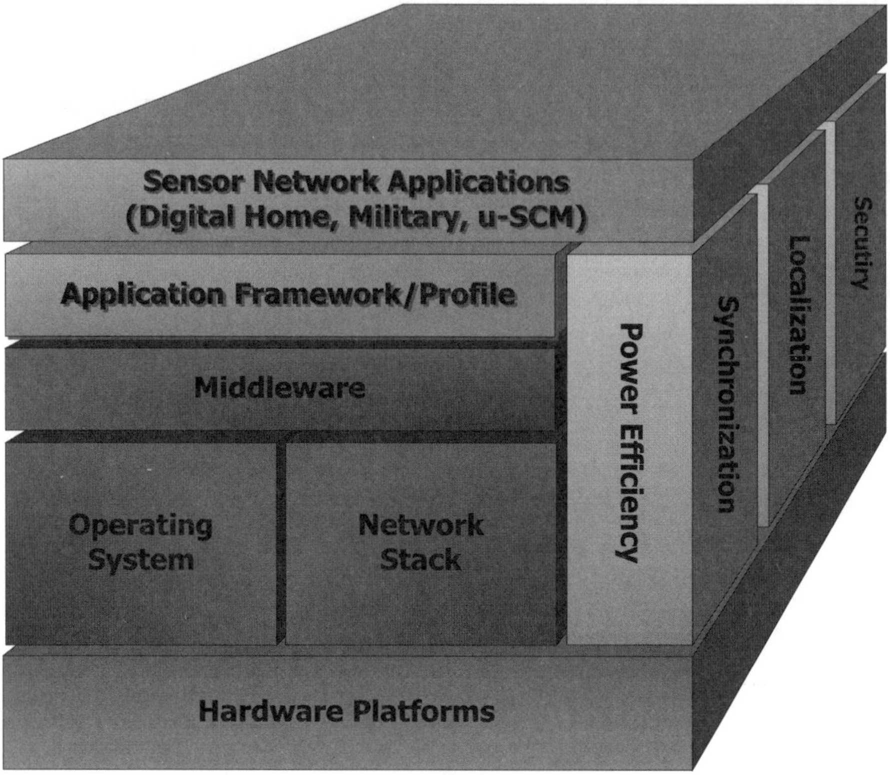

Fig. **10.** ANTS Architecture

In order to convey the data from wireless sensor networks at home to the Physio-Grid Network and to analyze and process the data, the project unified the wired and wireless networks. Moreover, investigations on distributed process and resource management were also made using lightweight grid technology and a user interface was developed for application services. The architecture is shown in Fig. 11.

The ANTS research team developed the sensor network field utilized in the project. In our work, the host attached to the ECG collector gets patient status information and forwards it to the sensor node. This sends the data to other sensor nodes across the sensor network via RF. Similarly, another host receives the data from the sensor network and forwards it to the server using TCP/IP.

Further sections will introduce part of our work in the ANTS architecture.

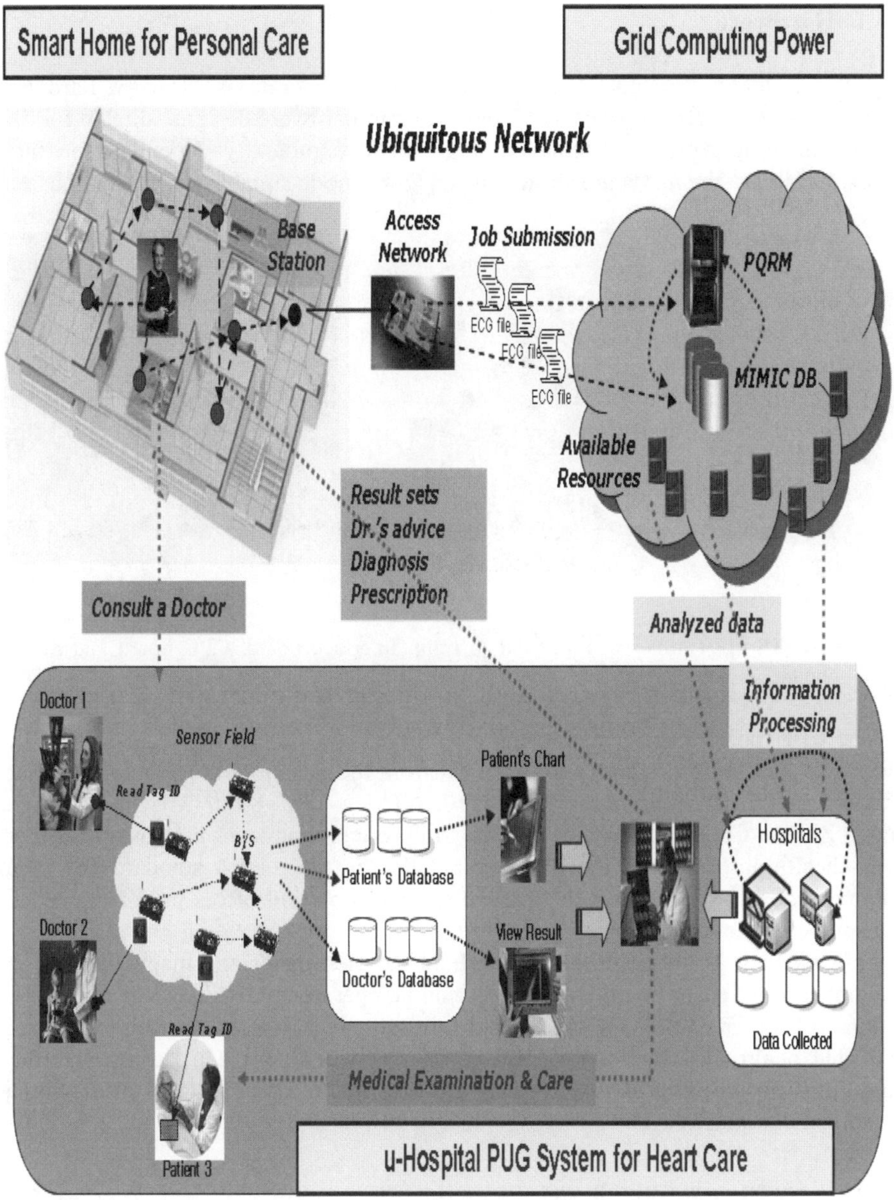

Fig. 11. E-Health Project Architecture

2.3.1 Hardware

ANTS architecture includes, besides software considerations, its own hardware support. Our system is comprised of four different hardware designs suitable for different sensor network requirements. It grows in complexity depending on their needs. In Fig. 12 the hardware shows an ANTS H2 node suitable for U-Healthcare.

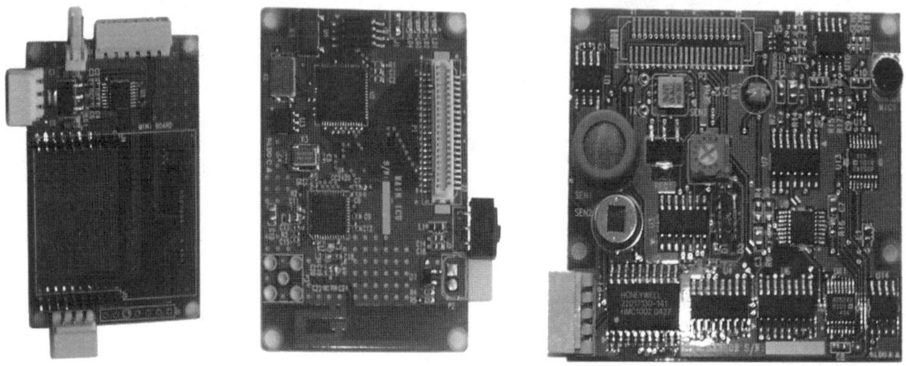

Fig. 12. ANTS H2 Hardware. From left to right, Interface board, CPU board and Sensor board

The CPU board is responsible for monitoring and processing signals from devices such as the ECG signal and heartbeat from the Sensor board. Some characteristics of the CPU board include an AMTEL ATMega128L 8 bit/8MHz µ-Controller and a Zigbee CC2420 transceiver. For wireless communication transmitting personal health information, the designs include the 802.11.5.4 standard for radio communication. It is used in the Zigbee specification and offers promising reductions in power consumption.

Sensors such as the ECG, heartbeat, light, accelerometer and magnetometer are integrated into Sensor board. All sensors can be operated individually or in collaboration with other sensors. If we want to use an external health sensor or transmit collected health information to local computer system, we can use an Interface board. It supports Serial/Parallel communication able to communicate with external sensors or computers.

2.3.2 ANTS Operating System

The ANTS Operating System (ANTS EOS) [16] is the core of this architecture and it coordinates the structural design in order to provide services which can evolve. With low-power consumption, small size code, small data size and an evolvable architecture as design criteria, we have developed this operating system for wireless sensor network applications. The EOS provides efficient memory space thread management, collaborative thread communication and a network stack. It also supports power management of the microcontroller and the radio transceiver, and a network wide time synchronization function. The most important feature of this OS is the concept that it can evolve. The operating system has features such as scalability, high-modularity. It is also able to upgrade during operating conditions. This is called "On-the-fly" upgradeability, that is, the operating system can be upgraded without interfering with user applications. The architecture of the EOS is shown in Fig. 13.

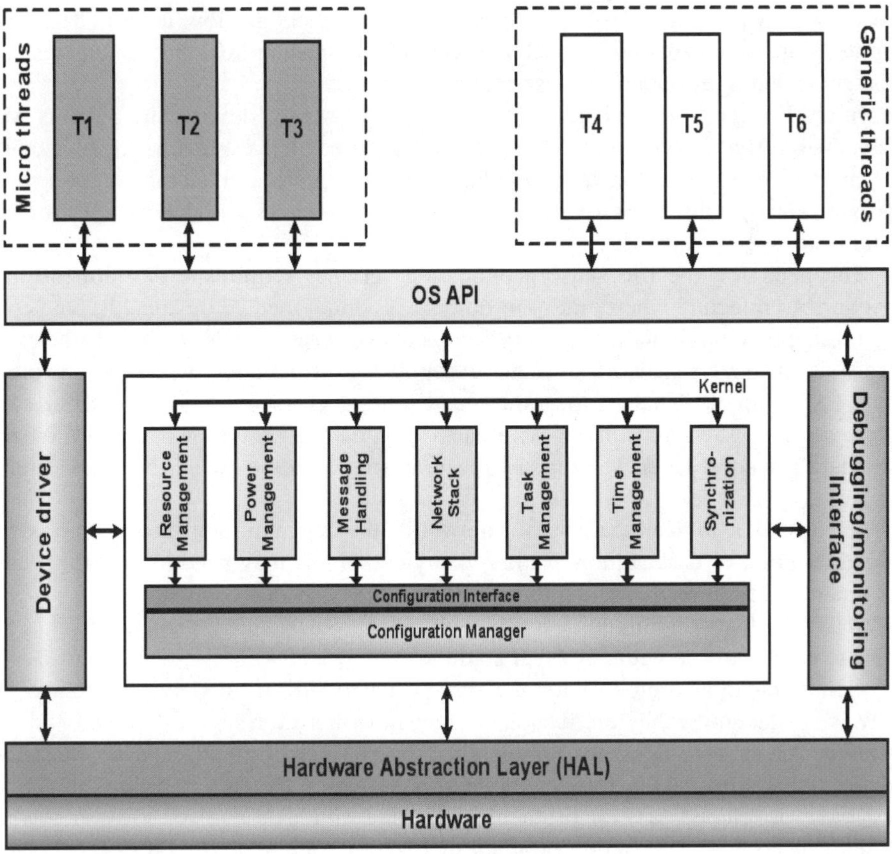

Fig. 13. ANTS EOS Architecture

2.3.3 Network Architecture and Protocols

The network architecture of ANTS is a two-tier, two-dimension (2T2D) network. This architecture supports various sensor nodes having different hardware capabilities and communication models for the support of various applications.

The two-tier network architecture supports sensor nodes with different hardware capabilities which include MCU (microcontroller unit), memory and sensors. ANTS currently supports two types of sensor nodes. One type operates as high performance sensor nodes which can for example provide time and location information references to other low-level sensor nodes by equipping high cost hardware devices such as GPS and high resolution oscillators. The others are low level nodes, with limited hardware capability, which operate only as sensing information sources and routers which relay data to its destination.

In the healthcare sensor networks, the types of sensor devices the patients will have, will differ according to the condition monitored. The caregivers may have different devices suitable for the particular patient. Network architecture support must provide for various types of sensor nodes. This is an essential design factor for healthcare sensor networks.

The need for specific sensor application services requires a two-dimensional network architecture where transport domain is complemented by an additional context or application domain necessary for exclusive services. ANTS defines the existence of an overlay network over the transport sensor networks which uses explicit network protocols. That is, location aimed routing protocols which can offer concrete services such as Context-Awareness beyond the limitations imposed by the standard transport layer, see Fig. 14 for an example on the ANTS Network Architecture.

In particular, in healthcare sensor networks, the destination of information is not a central point or base station. Rather, many caregivers may need to know the state of a particular patient. Unlike the conventional many-to-one communication system, a kind of multicast communication is required. In other words, all stations must be able to communicate with any other station.

Communication protocols for the transport network are of key importance for any WSN design as they are responsible for how the information is routed and delivered. As sensor nodes are principally powered with limited capacity batteries, work in this area usually focuses on energy efficiency for data transport. In ANTS we have developed several protocols with this aim. ANTS-PAD (Power Aware Data-centric) [19] is a routing protocol that achieves high energy efficiency by improving the MPEG (Minimum Energy Path Graph). PAD additionally supports the mobility of nodes and of self-healing when some nodes become inoperative. This is necessary to achieve optimum results by using hop count and power consumption values for metrics and minimizing packet delivery by being fully triggered. ANTS-PAC (Power Aware Chain) [17] is an energy efficient chain-based routing scheme that calculates transmission costs based on received signal strength and provides a

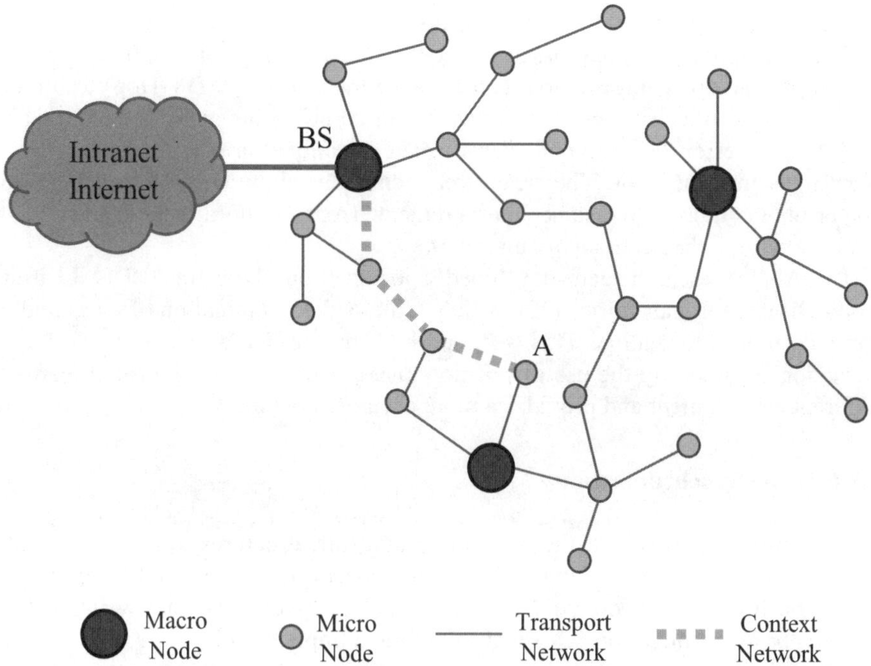

Fig. 14. ANTS Network Architecture

more prolonged network lifetime when compared with routing protocols. Finally ANTS-PPVR (Power-aware Position Vector Routing) is a protocol that provides optimum routes based on power information and location information. PPVR reduces the power consumption by using the Greedy Approach. It leads to a successful rate of packet delivery by avoiding void node area. That is regions characterized for being unreachable due to node communication being out of range.

The support for network mobility is also of great importance. This occurs mainly in situations where groups of nodes (patients) move freely but still require full connectivity. ANTS-SUMMA (Sub-network Mobility support with Multi-channel Assignment in wireless sensor network) [15] can support the sub-network mobility of the sensors. SUMMA achieves efficient packet transmission, robust interconnection and longer life-time with an efficient gateway election algorithm and data aggregation at gateway level.

Localization or position information is considered important for many WSN applications including a U-Healthcare system. When the health condition of the patient is monitored and a state of emergency occurs, the position of the patient and the health condition information is important for appropriate care.

Traditional approaches to the localization problem have employed position aware anchors, triangulation, range-based (using distance measurement, AHLoS) or range-free (using the other information than distance measurement, DV-Hop) techniques. The range-based techniques work well only in an environment with small distance measurement error and high node density. The techniques are de-pendent on the distance measurement error. The range-free techniques show con-stant average position errors in addition to distance measurement errors. In short, there is no single solution satisfying the accuracy requirement.

The ANTS research team developed a localization algorithm (LDL, Learning-based Distance Localization) [20], which exploits the combination of measured and non-measured information. This is, based both on measured distances and hop information obtained by the use of position aware anchors. The algorithm learns the different environment and provides a more accurate position.

2.3.4 Time Synchronization

Time information is one of the most important infrastructures to any collaborative system, such as the monitoring and tracking system. For an example, when we report some information on vital parameter and symptom, we may want to know 'when?' or 'how long?' or 'what is the combined implication?'.

Maintaining accurate time information in each system not only provides meaningful information, but also connects the system with our real physical world and can result in savings in energy or redundant information detection. For the saving in energy, a synchronized sensor can sleep for an amount of time, already promised with the monitoring sensor. To prevent redundancy, when more than two sensors detect the same event in an adjacent area we can filter out the redundancy.

Basically time synchronization can be applied when a system beings its activity and by synchronizing its clock to a reference clock. Local clocks of sensor network nodes are inherently inaccurate and prone to deviations of up to several seconds per week. To maintain network requirements in the order of micro-seconds, periodical synchronization of sensor nodes is required.

2.4 Concluding Remarks

In the new field of Wireless Sensor Networks, health monitoring services for medical care applications appear to be a promising research area with a wide range of possibilities. There are many challenges to overcome in developing future WSN applications. In this chapter we have introduced challenges and current research in U-Healthcare. We have also introduced ANTS as our solution for WSN in general and its healthcare applications in particular. We outlined some specific topics and have explained how our approach can effectively solve the problems. The ANTS research team will continue working on the WSN architecture to make the use of sensors a reality.

3 Real-time Health-Monitoring Network

3.1 Introduction

In the previous sections, we introduced the concept of ubiquitous healthcare and the Wireless Sensor Network (WSN). This section introduces the health monitoring sensor network based on the mobile Internet [21] as one of the future U-health services. We discuss the results from emulated implementation of a similar information network using the Mobile Web page as a WML health-information system. We assume the data transmission unit from the watch phone which is connected to the health-monitoring sensors. Our main interest is to determine whether the real-time information service is possible with an inexpensive Web server. We also consider which other factors should be considered for the implementation of a real-time health-monitoring sensor network. Particular interest is focused on the Web server at this center of the health-monitoring network.

3.2 Related Works

3.2.1 Related Works as Background

As an introduction, we have considered some related issues studied by other researchers concerning disabled and elderly people. First, we considered the results for the disabled and elderly people resulting from our R&D projects. It is desirable to introduce the successful products or services now available for universal access. Universal access implies the accessibility and usability of Information Society Technologies (IST) by anyone, anywhere at anytime. Research and Development in IT now prove its impact on the quality of life of the target groups [22]. To fail to involve consumers in the process of matching the person and the assistive technology perpetuates a system of service delivery that has not been as effective as it could be from both the outcome achievement and marketplace perspective. This is discussed in the study of assistive technology outcomes in the United States by Scherer [23].

We have discussed the U-healthcare as well as WSN (Wireless Sensor Network) in the previous sections. Investigations for the disabled and elderly have been advanced recently by many researchers. The mobile phone based user interface concept for health data acquisition at home was studied by Schreier et al. [24], especially using the camera-phone for photographing the measured health-data. An adaptive interface based upon biofeedback sensors was studied by Velasco et al. [25]. They are investigating applications in the area of computing and multimodal interfaces using wireless sensors and roaming profiles. A com-puter-based self-health monitoring system for the elderly living in a low income housing environment was studied by Karshmer [26]. The key finding is that information technology and a well designed user interface can be a valuable supplement to traditional healthcare.

For the visually impaired in an educational environment, the use of the bar code and the RFID with a reader-writer attached to a PDA was studied by Tatsumi et al. [27] as a promising step toward building an information ensured area. This was especially relevant to obtain information from a bar code or from RFID tags attached to equipment or surroundings.

'Smart environments for all' was the theme introduced to the session by Nussbaum [28]. He stressed that smart environments have the potential to increase the quality as well as the efficiency of healthcare. Development of smart home technologies for people with disabilities provides a challenge to determine accurate requirements and needs in dynamic situations. Feki et al. [29] introduced the integration of context awareness and multimodal functionalities in the smart environment. Information such as the availability of resources, user profiles, location, input controls and services can be used to improve the interaction between users and their environments.

New approaches and related instruments are needed for capturing human requirements in the new conditions. An appropriate architectural framework and development tools will need to be elaborated in the age of the disappearing computer [30]. The development of highly efficient and effective user interfaces, which are matched to the user needs and abilities, was discussed for the successful application of assistive technology [31]. We are mainly concerned with the mobile health-monitoring device and the health-monitoring network in the future. We can consider the usage of information with voice interface in the near future. Pervasive healthcare would improve the productivity of healthcare practitioners and greatly facilitate the delivery of a wider range of medical services [32]. In order to enhance the quality of life for people with disabilities and of elderly people who need to be independent the integration of networking and communication technologies in the smart home concept dedicated to people with disabilities was studied by Ghorbel et al. [33]. Computing and mobile applications are key technologies that may help them to remain at home. Giroux et al. [34] introduced the concept of an infrastructure using indoor computing and outdoor mobile computing in order to provide assistance and tele-monitoring.

3.2.2 Related Works for Performance

The existance of the World-Wide Web (WWW) servers is a central factor in the provision of ubiquitous, reliable, and efficient information. The performance issues in Web servers were studied [35]. We discuss performance considerations of the health-monitoring network using an inexpensive Web server for healthcare of the disabled and elderly people. We discuss the issues concerning the performance of the mobile Internet environment and consider the implementation. For the mobile Internet, the WAP protocol [36] has been frequently used especially in Korea and other countries. WAP browsers, versions 1.0 and 2.0, have also been implemented in many mobile phone devices.

Several studies by several researchers are now introduced. These consider the performance in the wired and the mobile Internet. A new performance analysis methodology for health-monitoring services in the area of pervasive and ubiquitous computing is needed. The wireless, mobile Web promises to provide users with unrestricted access to information. This will also aid acceptance of new services that are specialized for mobile use [38]. For health monitoring services, we need to consider the performance of the user interface for the disabled. We should consider Quality of Service (QoS), and the speed of real-time health monitoring services will be one of the most important qualities. New performance analysis methodologies for information networks, based on the disabled user's perspective were studied. We introduce analysis for real-time unified portals for an information network based on wired and mobile Internet.

We now discuss the performance, constraints and analysis, and consider the requirements for performance in the pervasive computing environment.

The difficulties in simulating the Internet were discussed by Floyd and Faxson [40]. Factors which must be considered are now discussed. The heterogeneity of the network and the rapid change of traffic depending upon new applications, the Web environment and the stochastic characteristics of the session arrivals and connection sizes. Here, traffic behavior needs to have deterministic characteristics instead of having the heavy tailed distribution of the related random variables. This includes the arrival rate, transmission time of packets through Internet, processing times of the server, and the size of the contents of health-monitoring information. Barford and Crovella [41] studied the critical path analysis of TCP transactions as follows. Previous work in performance analysis and the improvement of Web transactions fall into two categories. These are the work on servers, and work on networks and protocols. These works studied the effects of file size, server load, network load, path length, and the causes of variability in transfer duration. The conclusion is that the server load is the major determiner of transfer time for small files, while network load is the major determiner for large files. In addition, the dominant cause of variability in transfer time is packet loss. From the results of this research, it appears that to minimize the dependency of the overall performance of the health-monitoring to the network traffic we should use very small files for health-monitoring data. That is, WML Web page for mobile Internet and HTML page for wired Internet. The number of packets for one transaction should be as small as possible. For small sized file or Web page, the sever load is the major factor in determining the performance of health-monitoring. Therefore the server should be dedicated to a single purpose. This is, it should be used for the dedicated health-monitoring Web server.

3.3 Health-Monitoring Sensors and Network

Various type of health monitoring sensors for real application in the future can be considered. Here we consider the wrist phone as one of the future products to measure health data, the pulse at wrist, the blood pressure, the strength of pulse, for example. Because oriental medical science is using this information in the wrist to diagnose personal health, even although that information may not be exact for health diagnosis. Health-monitoring sensors will become more accurate and easier to use. This is based on the U-health technologies discussed in the previous subsections and on the evolution of MEMS (Micro Electronic Mechanical System) and USN (Ubiquitous Sensor Network) technologies.

3.3.1 Health-Monitoring Sensors in the Wrist Phone

Figure 15 shows health-monitoring sensors in the wrist phone on the hand of the disabled and elderly people. The wrist phone is a future product not yet implemented. We assume that the sensors for the pulse, the strength of the pulse, and blood pressure would provide raw data about health of the person.

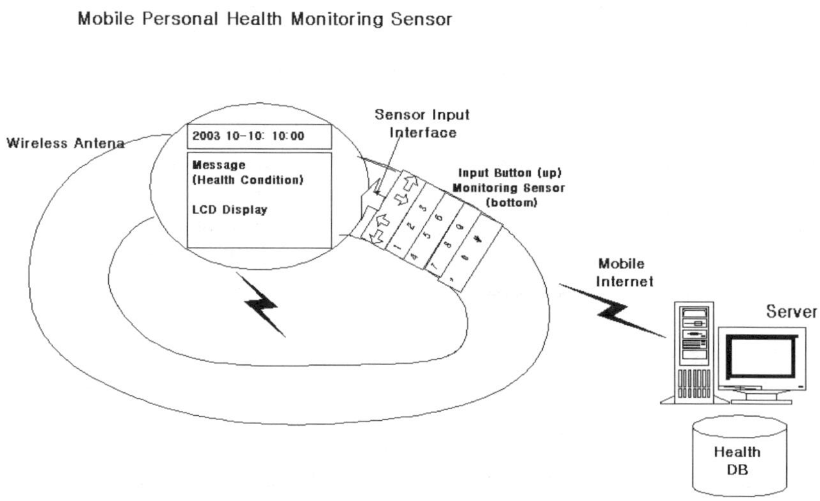

Fig. 15. Mobile Health-Monitoring Sensors based on the use of the Wrist Phone

Glitho et al. [42] provided a case study on mobile agents and their use for information retrieval; the following health-monitoring sensors on wrist phones may be considered as mobile agents even though they are not for the same applications. Here instead of a plain client-server, we need an optimized client server or the mobile agent approach for use of our health-monitoring sensor network with the health Web server.

The performance analysis for the real-time health monitoring system may be different from the conventional analysis methodologies of non-real-time applications. We should investigate this new approach, because the real-time health-monitoring network may be applicable to many new applications for the disabled and elderly in pervasive healthcare. We studied the real-time health-monitoring application, frequently getting personal information. This was in addition to written information frequently getting personal information. This was in addition to written information provided by clients or health-monitoring agents.

3.3.2 Health-Monitoring Network

For the real-time health-monitoring network using mobile Internet, shown in Fig. 16, the dominating factor and the deviation of the variable should be within the available response time. To be deterministic in the real-time application, the estimation time should be bounded within deterministic time. The interchange of data between the watch phone and the server should be automatic except where information is requested by the user. The Web server should be efficient and have high performance in the dedicated application. The data exchanged and analyzed information should be as simple as possible and have a simplified efficient format. If possible, the bandwidth requirement for wireless or mobile Internet should be immune to network traffic conditions. That is also desirable with respect to the degradation caused by the other services sharing the same network and server.

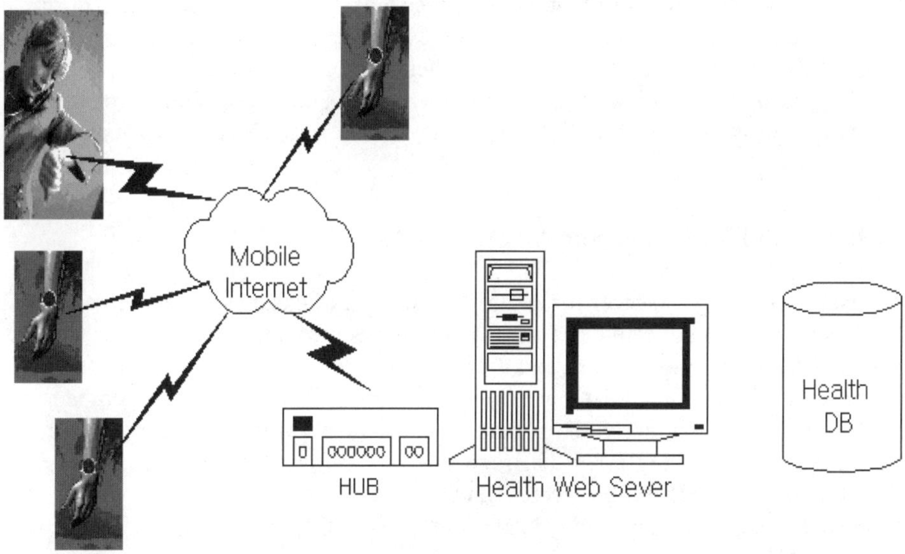

Fig. 16. Mobile Health-Monitoring Network

The time spent in the Web server may be considered to be immune to the network and server condition. In short packets below 1.5Kbytes that may be the upper bound of packet size. In general, the frequency of health monitoring is greater than a frequency of the analyzed or diagnosed information obtained from the health Web server. This system is based on wired or mobile Internet. The monitored health data from sensors in a watch phone can be registered at any time using the mobile Internet with the domain name of test Web server. That is, 'ktrip.net' [43] for wired/mobile Internet. This site has been used as a real-time information network server and we considered it as a health-monitoring server because it can be used as a Web server for testing.

3.4 Health Information Server

An information center designed to meet the needs of people with disabilities will help them to achieve a higher degree of independence and facilitate their integration into the community. The following four perspectives, discussed by Kowalik [44], ensure that a particular disability will not prevent the use of the information system. For a disabled person to fully use the information stored in the information system's database, they have to be able to successfully complete four tasks: 1. Connect to the information system; 2. Say exactly what information they need; 3. Receive the requested information; 4. Record it in a way that will allow multiple use of the information.

Several factors need to be considered when providing for health information. These include the following factors. 1. Consistency of health-monitoring information ; 2. Convenient user interface; 3. Universal access and universal design for the disabled and elderly people; 4. A unified health-monitoring Web server for wired Internet and mobile Internet. 5. Health-information center accessibility for the doctor nurse, and the disabled and elderly; 6. Provision for different formats of health information.

3.4.1 Health Information and Analysis Model

We used a single Web server for health information to ensure for cost-effectiveness and simplicity of management. This offers effectiveness and efficiency for the real-time health-monitoring network and the utilization of resources.

We assume that the wrist phone with health-monitoring sensors provides the health information regularly. This must be chosen carefully and is a matter for further research. Depending upon the frequency of writing the health information, the workload of the health Web server will change. The interval of regular writing may be considered as an arrival rate in the queuing performance analysis model. The transmission packet unit for billing by mobile communication service provider is about 0.5 Cents (U.S.); for a packet size of 512 Bytes. This is the minimum packet size for billing in Korea. If possible, the health-monitoring data for the wrist phone to the server through mobile Internet should be less than 512 Bytes. This is further bounded to be much below 1.5Kbytes. The further boundary will be discussed later. A SMS (Short Message Service) data, which consists of 80 Bytes, costs around 2.5 Cents (U.S.) in Korea. The WML packet cost is much lower than an SMS message in terms of cost.

3.4.2 Health Information Web Server

The health Web server should have the capability to show the appropriate health contents. That is, the HTML contents for the wired Internet in addition to the mobile contents of many different kinds of mobile devices, for example WML, mHTML, HDML. For the unified service, there are several constraints when compared to wired Internet. We should consider various kinds of mobile devices browsers for the mobile Internet. Each of those devices may have different image capabilities. The development and application is very different to the existing wired Internet. That is why it is mainly based on the almost unified browser, MS Explorer. We considered only text-based health-monitoring information from the wrist phone to the heath-monitoring Web server and vice versa. This is in order to be immune to any type of Internet traffic load and to minimize the mobile communication cost of health-monitoring services.

We suggest to provide the minimum requirements for the wired Internet with a PC and for the mobile Internet using the wireless mobile devices. For example, handheld devices and mobile phones can provide the simplest functionality compared with the less capable mobile Internet phones. Among the several constraints with the mobile phone, the WML deck size should be below 1.5 Kbyte. We implemented a similar Web Server Information Network for the wired Internet using a PC for the wireless Internet with mobile devices. We consider the Web server as a health information Web server. The size of contents is below 1.5Kbyte as a WML deck, which is the transmission packet unit in the WAP environment. Even for the wired Internet we considered for health information services the same content with a small size of Web page.

3.4.3 Emulated Implementation and Empirical Results

The implemented system is as follows is a leased E1 (2.048 Mbps) Internet communication line to a router and to test Web server. That is, the health-monitoring web server for both wired and mobile Internet is used. As we have already discussed, the size of Web page for a unified service was considered to be below 1.5Kbyte for monitored health data and information. 5Kbytes of the almost same analyzed or diagnosed information for wired PC Internet, to minimize the dependency of the overall performance to the shared and stochastically varying network traffic. The Web server is dedicated to minimize the server load and is dedicated to the health-monitoring network.

From the mean and standard deviation determined from 100 samples using the emulated health-monitoring Web server, we see that the response time of the wired PC is the fastest and most stable with little deviation. The average response time with mobile phone Internet is about 12 seconds with a 2 second standard deviation. The other two cases with wired PC via the intermediate server show that, depending upon the intermediate server, the mean and deviation of the response time are very different. The size of Web page for the wired Internet accessed by the domain name ktrip.net is about 5 Kbytes, and the size of the mobile Web page is about 1.5Kbytes. This becomes about 1Kbytes after compiling to WAP binary file. That is considered as health information. The mobile 1.5Kbyte content retrieval time with mobile Internet is about 10 seconds longer than the wired (PC) 5Kbyte content retrieval time due to the elapsed time with the gateway and base station. This is the time which should be considered for health-monitoring applications with the mobile Internet.

We are able to make the processing time dependent on the Web server. It is determined by the size of the packet. It can be considered as a queuing model with a Markovian arrival rate (M). It has a deterministic processing time with departure rate (D).

3.5 Concluding Remarks and Future Works

A real-time health-monitoring network for disabled and elderly people, using the domain name 'ktrip.net', has been studied on the basis of a wired and a mobile Internet. The results of implementation show that the overhead time in the mobile Internet is not negligible for a real-time health-monitoring network. The evaluation of the health-monitoring Web server for the wired and mobile Internet can be applied to provide an efficient investment for worldwide health-monitoring services. For future work, the availability of the health Web server will be studied in terms of the reliability of the health-monitoring sensor network. Also, a meaningful parameter for analyzing and diagnosing personal health will be studied. This will be based on the research U-healthcare and WSN discussed in the previous subsections for real-time monitoring.

References

1. Pattichis CS. et al.: Wireless telemedicine system. An Overview, IEEE Antenna and Propagation Magazine, 44(2), pp. 143-153, 2002.
2. Yoo SK. et al.: Prototype design of mobile emergency telemedicine system, LNCS 3481, pp. 1028-1034, 2005.
3. Budinger TF: Biomonitoring with wireless communications. Annu. Rev. Biomed. Eng., 5, PP.383-412, 2003.
4. Yoo SK et al.: Design of a PC-based multimedia telemedicine system for baring function teleconsultation. Int. J. of Medical Informatics. 61, pp. 217-227, 2001.
5. Yoo SK et al.: Real-time emergency telemedicine system: Prototype design and functional evaluation. Yonsei Medical J., 45(3), pp. 501-509, 2004.
6. Kim BS, Yoo SK: Motion artifact reduction in Photoplesthmography using independent component analysis, 2005. (in Press).

7. Istepanian RSH. Pertrosian A.: Optimal Zonal Wavelet-based ECG Data Compression for Mobile Telecardiology System. IEEE trans. Inform. Technol. Biomed, 4, pp. 200-211, 2000.
8. A. Mainwaring, J. Polastre, R. Szewczyk, D. Culler and J. Anderson: Wireless Sensor Networks for Habitat Monitoring, WSNA'02, September 28, Atlanta, Georgia, USA, 2002.
9. T. Liu and M. Martonosi: Impala: A Middleware System for Managing Autonomic Sensor Systems, Computer Science. Princeton University.
10. D. Wang, E. Arens, T. Webster and M. Shi: How The Number And Placement Of Sensors Controlling Room Air Distribution Systems Affect Energy Use And Comfort, Center for Environmental Design Research, University of California, Berkeley.
11. M. Srivastava, R. Muntz, M. Potkonjak: Smart Kindergarten: Sensor-based Wireless Networks for Smart Developmental Problem-solving Environments, ACM SIGMOBILE 7/01 Rome, Italy.
12. J. Hill, R. Szewczyk, A. Woo, S. Hollar, D. Culler and K. Pister: System Architecture Directions for Networked Sensors, ASPLOS IX, November 2000, Cambridge, MA, USA.
13. Konrad Lorincz *et al*: Sensor Networks for emergency respone, IEEE pervasive computing, pp. 16-23, 2004.
14. Emil Jovanov, Aleksandar Milenkovic, Chris Otto and Piet C de Groen: A wireless body area network of intelligent motion sensors for computer assisted physical rehabilitation, Journal of NeuroEngineering and Rehabilitation 2005.
15. J. Park, D. Kim: SUMMA: Sub-network Mobility support using Multi-channel Assignment in wireless sensor networks, Master Thesis, School Engineering, Information and Communications University 2005.
16. T. Do, D. Kim, T. Sanchez, H. Kim, S. Hong, M. Pham, K. Lee, S. Park: An Evolvable Operating System for Wireless Sensor Networks, to appear in International Embedded and Hybrid Systems Conference, Singapore, May. 10-May 13, 2005.
17. M. Pham, D. Kim, Y. Doh, S. Yoo: Power Aware Chain Routing Protocol for Data Gathering in Sensor Networks, to appear in IEEE International Conference on Intelligent Sensors, Sensor Networks & Information Processing, Australia, Dec. 14-17, 2004.
18. H. Song, D. Kim: Sensor Network Management System using UPnP, KISS Fall Conference, Oct. 2004.
19. N. Park, D. Kim, Y. Doh, S. Lee and J. Kim: Power Aware Data-centric Routing Protocol for Sensor Networks, Submitted to SCCI'05.
20. D. Bach and D. Kim: A Localization Algorithm Extension for The Evolvable Sensor Network, PDCS 2004, Cambridge, MA, USA.
21. Yung Bok Kim and Jong Yong Kim. Real-Time Health-Monitoring Network for Disabled and Elderly People. ICCHP 2004, LNCS 3118, pp. 377-384, 2004.
22. Christian Buhler: From Research to Business Improving the Take Up of Results of Research Projects. ICCHP 2002, LNCS 2398, pp. 6-7, 2002.
23. Marcia J. Scherer: The Study of Assistive Technology Outcomes in the United States. ICCHP 2002, LNCS 2398, pp. 764-771, 2002.

24. Gunter Schreier, Alexander Kollmann, Martin Kramer, Jurgen Messmer, Andreas Hochgatterer, and Peter Kastner. Mobile Phone Based User Interface Concept for Health data Acquisition at Home. ICCHP 2004, LNCS3118, pp. 29-36, 2004.
25. Carlos A. Velasco, Yehya Mohamad, Dirk Stegemann, Henrike Gappa, Gaby Nordbrock, Erwin Hartsuiker, Javier Sanchez-Lacuesta, and Juan M. Belda. IPCA: Adaptive Interfaces Based upon Biofeedback Sensors. ICCHP 2004, LNCS 3118, pp. 129-134, 2004.
26. Judith F. Karshmer and Arthur I. Karshmer. A Computer-Based Self-health Monitoring System for the Elderly Living in a Low Income Housing Environment. ICCHP 2004, LNCS 3118, pp. 385-391, 2004.
27. Hisayuki Tatsumi, Yasuyuki Murai, Masahiro Miyakawa, and Shinji Tokumasu. Use of Bar Code and RFID for the Visually Impaired in Educational Environment. ICCHP 2004, LNCS 3118, pp. 583-588, 2004.
28. Gerhard Nussbaum. Smart Environments for All Introduction to the Special Thematic Session. ICCHP 2004, LNCS 3118, pp. 889-890, 2004.
29. Mohamed Ali Feki, Stephane Renouard, Bessam Abdulrazak, Gerard Chollet, and Mounir Mokhtari. Coupling Context Awareness and Multimodality in Smart Homes Concept. ICCHP 2004, LNCS 3118, pp. 906-913, 2004.
30. Constantine Stephanidis: The Disappearing Computer: Emerging Opportunities and Challenges for Disables and Elderly People. ICCHP 2002, LNCS 2398, pp. 41-48, 2002.
31. Wolfgang L. Zagler: Matching Typing Person and Intelligent Interfaces. ICCHP 2002, LNCS 2398, pp. 241-242, 2002.
32. Upkar Varshney: Pervasive Healthcare. Computer, December, pp. 138-140, 2003.
33. Mahmoud Ghorbel, Maria-Teresa Segarra, Jerome Kerdreux, Ronan Keryell, Andre Thepaut, Mounir Mokhtari. Networking and Communication in Smart Home for People with Disabilities. ICCHP 2004, LNCS 3118, pp. 937-944, 2004.
34. Sylvain Giroux, Helene Pigot, and Andre Mayers. Indoors Pervasive Computing and Outdoors Mobile Computing for Cognitive Assistance and Telemonitoring. ICCHP 2004, LNCS 3118, pp. 953-960, 2004.
35. Erich Nahum, Tsipora Barzilai, and Dilip D. Kandlur: Performance Issues in WWW Servers. IEEE/ACM Transactions on Networking, vol. 10, no. 1, February, pp. 2-11, 2002.
36. Vijay Kumar, Srinivas Parimi and Dharma P. Agrawal: WAP: Present and Future. IEEE Pervasive Computing, January-March, pp. 79-83, 2003.
37. Yih-Farn Robin Chen and Charles Petrie: Ubiquitous Mobile Computing. IEEE Internet Computing, March-April, pp. 16-17, 2003.
38. Ariel Pashtan, Shriram Kollipara and Michael Pearce. Adapting Content for Wireless Web Services. IEEE Internet Computing. September-October, pp. 79-85, 2003.
39. Yung Bok Kim and Jong Yong Kim. Performance Analysis of User Interface for the Disabled in Real-Time Ubiquitous Information Network. ICCHP 2004, LNCS 3118, pp. 926-929, 2004.

40. Sally Floyd and Vern Paxson: Difficulties in Simulating the Internet. IEEE/ACM Transactions on Networking, vol.9, no.4, August, pp. 392-403, 2001.
41. Paul Barford and Mark Crovella: Critical Path Analysis of TCP Transactions. IEEE/ACM Transactions on Networking, vol.9, no.3, June, pp. 238-248, 2001.
42. Roch H. Glitho, Edgar Olougouna and Samuel Pierre: Mobile Agents and Their Use for Information Retrieval: A Brief Overvies and an Elaborate Case Study. IEEE Network, January/February, pp. 34-41, 2002.
43. Real-time Information Network site for Health-monitoring Emulation (Mobile/wired Web Site) http://ktrip.net
44. Ryszard Kowalik. Capabilities and Limitations of the Disabled in Remote Access to Information. ICCHP 2002, LNCS 2398, pp. 707-708, 2002.

2 Multimedia Medical Informatics System in Healthcare

Cecília Sik Lányi
Faculty of Information Technology,
University of Veszprém
H-8200 Veszprém, Egyetem u. 10., Hungary

Abstract. In our modern 21st century, daily life would be unthinkable without computers. Multimedia and virtual reality are useful for people with spe-

in medical informatics, rehabilitation and assistive & preventive healthcare. This chapter deals with multimedia applications intended for use by medical doctors, nurses and other interested persons. It describes ways in which multimedia can assist in their work. These include the areas of diagnosis and the application to training. Matters that are important to patients are also dealt with. Some of these are how multimedia can help their rehabilitation.

1. Introduction

This chapter deals with multimedia applications intended for use by medical doctors, nurses and other interested persons. It describes ways in which multimedia can assist in their work. These include the areas of diagnosis and the application to training. Matters that are important to patients are also dealt with. Some of these are how multimedia can help their rehabilitation. It is especially beneficial to those who suffer from asthma, low vision, hearing problems, are aphasic or had a stroke. Other uses of multimedia, such as in the rehabilitation of dyslexic or autistic persons are not discussed in this chapter. It is necessary to begin with some appropriate definitions.

1.1. What is Multimedia?

Multimedia refers to the use of computers to present text, graphics, animation, and sound in an integrated way. Long heralded as the future revolution in computing, multimedia applications were, until the mid-90s, uncommon due to the expensive hardware required. With increases in computer performance and decreases in price, however, multimedia is now commonplace. Nearly all PCs are capable of displaying video, though the resolution available depends on the power of the computer's video adapter and CPU.

C.S. Lányi: *Multimedia Medical Informatics System in Healthcare*, Studies in Computational Intelligence (SCI) **19**, 37–86 (2006)
www.springerlink.com

The term multimedia describes a number of diverse technologies that allow visual and audio media to be combined in new ways for the purpose of communicating. Applications include entertainment, education and advertising. Multimedia often refers to computer technologies. Nearly every PC built today is capable of multimedia because they include a CD-ROM or DVD drive, and a good sound and video card (often built into the motherboard). But the term multimedia also describes a number of dedicated media appliances, such as digital video recorders (DVRs), interactive television, MP3 players, advanced wireless devices and public video displays [1]. In recent years, the term multimedia has taken on many diverse meanings for an ever-increasing audience. Some of us have a form of multimedia "narrowcast" through digital cable. Home DVD editing software can be categorized as multimedia, along with the latest generation of mobile phones which are capable of taking and sending voice annotated photos. The term multimedia will continue to evolve and will take on as many new meanings as the technologies and applications it is being used to describe. From our viewpoint multimedia is a means of communication that combines text with graphics, sound, animation, full-motion video, etc. - usually in a highly interactive way, and it also includes the use of the Internet.

1.2. What is the assistive and preventive healthcare?

Assistive and adaptive technologies can enhance the lives of individuals with disabilities. It can increase their independence and productivity, and help them gain greater social inclusion. However, the meaning of "Assistive Technology" often remains unclear and fuzzy to many healthcare professionals and the disabled people who could benefit from it. Preventive in medical terms is a prophylactic action, preventing or slowing the course of an illness or a disease. It includes also the treatment and management of illness and the preservation of mental and physical well-being through the services offered by the medical and allied health professions. Using multimedia in the assistive and preventive healthcare is sphere discussed in this chapter.

2. Background

Multimedia applications are used by physicians, nurses and patients. The healthcare staff use multimedia applications for saving and sending images. Multimedia helps them make diagnoses. It is also used for medical education, training and teleconferencing. Patients use multimedia as an informatics tool in their education and rehabilitation. The main question is how can we develop these multimedia applications? How can the user's needs and the technical possibilities be harmonised?

The vision of Morris in 1999 was that by the year 2008, a major reorganization of health care services in the United States would have evolved from the previous solo- and group-practice models of the 1940s. These include fee-for-service, insurer-indemnification financing, paper-based information systems, to nationwide managed care plans employing enhanced computer-based information systems [2]. This vision is partly true, but we are still far from the global use of multimedia and of the Internet.

The origin of medical record writing goes back to Hippocrates and over many centuries this important medical duty has been regarded as an annoying, laborious and error-prone task. First steps towards better medical record taking and archiving started in 1936 with punch cards. In the 1960s the minimum basic data set, a unique patient ID, was introduced and, even for outpatients the first computerized medical record systems were developed using some important standards and well accepted data structures. Nowadays multimedia are included in patient record systems, and highly specialized subsystems such as those for radiology or cardiology are available. Semantic and data mining techniques as well as medical classifications and standardized terminologies support the evaluation. These methods should improve the quality of care, reduce errors, improve communication between multiple specialists. It should also reduce waiting times for patients and improve efficiency. Over decades it has become obvious that the structure of a medical record, notably for coded data but also for narrative text and pictures, must be carefully modelled. Well maintained standardized health terminologies and medical classifications are important issues for a user-friendly electronic medical record [3].

2.1 Examples of multimedia healthcare informatics applications

The definition of health information is growing to include multimedia audio, video, and high-resolution still images. Many image-processing applications, handling medical images, have been developed all over the world. Telemedicine is one example. At East Carolina University School of Medicine a program including the telemedicine applications presently in use was implemented and the virtual reality applications are currently under development. Included are the major design criteria that shape the telemedicine network. Some of the lessons learned in developing the network, and a discussion of the future of telemedicine are included. The incorporation of telemedicine within a fully integrated health information system as described by Balch and Tichenor [4] are considered. The use of digital medical images has become common over the last few years, coincident with the availability of inexpensive, mega-pixel quality digital cameras and the transition to digital radiology operation by hospitals. One problem that clinicians, medical educators, and basic scientists encounter when handling images is the difficulty of using business and graphic arts commercial-off-the-shelf (COTS) software in multicontext authoring and interactive teaching environments [5]. At the University of Utah scientists are investigating and developing software-supported methodologies to help clinicians, medical educators, and basic scientists. Goede and co-workers developed an annotation methodology that functions as a foundation for creating, using, reusing, and extending dynamic annotations in a context-appropriate, interactive digital environment. The annotation methodology supports the authoring process as well as output and presentation mechanisms. The annotation methodology is the foundation for a Windows implementation that allows annotated elements to be represented as structured eXtensible Markup Language and stored separately from the image(s).

A basic domain of medical imaging is anatomy. Therefore, anatomical knowledge is a rational basis for organizing and analysing images. The goals of the Digital Anatomist Program at the University of Washington include the development of an anatomically based software framework for organizing, analysing, visualizing and utilizing biomedical information [6].

At the University of Pittsburgh Medical Center images are stored in the Image Engine multimedia medical record system. This is enabled by an automated semantic indexing of radiology imaging. The authors used the SAPHIRE indexing system to automatically identify important biomedical concepts within radiology reports and represent these concepts with terms from the 1998 edition of the U.S. National Library of Medicine's Unified Medical Language System (UMLS) Metathesaurus. This automated UMLS indexing was then compared with manual UMLS indexing of the same reports. Human indexing identified appropriate UMLS. The overall conclusions of this pilot study were that the UMLS metathesaurus provided adequate coverage of the majority of the important concepts contained within the radiology report test set and that SAPHIRE could automatically identify and translate almost two thirds of these concepts into appropriate UMLS descriptors. Further work is required to improve both the recall and precision of this automated concept extraction process [7].

Prefetching methods have traditionally been used to restore archived images from picture archiving and communication systems to diagnostic imaging workstations prior to an anticipated need. This facilitates timely comparison of historical studies and patient management. Bui et al. [8] described a problem-oriented prefetching scheme, which details a mechanism supporting the selection of patients for prefetching via characterizations of clinical problems. It uses multiple data sources (picture archiving and communication systems, hospital information systems, and radiology information systems). Patients are classified into cohorts on the basis of their medical conditions (e.g., lung cancer); and prefetching of multimedia data (imaging, laboratory, and medical reports) from clinical databases. This enables an integrated patient record to be viewed. Preliminary evaluation of the prefetching algorithm using classic information retrieval measures showed that the system had high recall (100 percent), correctly identifying and retrieving data for all patients belonging to a target cohort, but it had a low precision (50 percent). A key finding during the testing was that the recall of the system was increased through the use of multiple data sources when compared with only one data source. This is because of better patient descriptors. Medical problems and patient cohorts were more specifically defined by combining information from heterogeneous databases.

It is clear that a comprehensive data warehouse framework is needed, which encompasses imaging and non-imaging information in supporting disease management and research. Stephen and co-workers propose such a framework, describing general design principles and system architecture. They illustrate a multimodality neuro-imaging data warehouse system implemented for clinical epilepsy research [9]. The data warehouse system is built on top of a picture archiving and communication system (PACS) environment and it applies an iterative object-oriented analysis and design (OOAD) approach and recognized data interface and design standards. The implementation is based on a Java CORBA (Common Object Request Broker Architecture) and Web-based architecture that separates the graphical user interface presentation, data warehouse business services, data staging area, and backend source systems into distinct software layers. The image data warehouse framework can be modified and generalized for new application domains

2.2 Establish diagnosis

Human event-related incidents reflect cognitive processing. They are normally elicited by external events, such as acoustic sounds or visual stimuli. As such they provide an opportunity to study normal and abnormal brain function non-invasively, at sub-second resolution. Advances in multimedia technology permit specialists in informatics and neuropsychology to cooperate in the design and implementation of paradigms, which influence ERP components. At the University of Ulster and the National University of Singapore the researchers illustrated the progression from standard paradigms to visual paradigms which can be used to study cognitive and emotional responses. Data from a study investigating the comparative processing of target pictures and words illustrate how external stimuli influence the later cognitive potentials [10].

Desmond and co-workers described a new system that scans electronic records from cardiac surgery and uses inference rules to identify and classify abnormal events (for example hypertension) that may occur during critical surgical points such as the start of bypass. This vital information is used as the content of automatically generated briefings designed by MAGIC, a multimedia system that they have developed to brief intensive care unit clinicians on patient status after cardiac surgery. By recognizing patterns in the patient record, they concisely summarize detailed patient data [11].

At the Myongji University and the Seoul National University (Korea) a medical teleconferencing system was designed and integrated with a multimedia patient database. It incorporated easy-to-use tools and functions to effectively support collaborative work between physicians in remote locations. The design provided a virtual workspace that allows physicians to collectively view various kinds of patient data. By integrating the teleconferencing function into this workspace, physicians were able to conduct conferences using the same interface and to have real-time access to the database during conference sessions [12].

2.3 The WEB and the mobile phones

The technical advances in Internet-based client/server applications and new multimedia communications protocols enable the development of cost-effective, platform-independent solutions to the problem of remote access to continuously acquired physiological data. The UCLA Neurosurgery Intensive Care Unit (ICU) has developed a distributed computer sys-tem that provides access over the World Wide Web (WWW) to current and previously acquired physiological data. This includes intracranial pressure, cerebral perfusion pressure, and heart rate from critical care patients. Physicians and clinical researchers can access the data through personal computers from their offices, from their homes, or even while on the road [13].

Another interesting project was the Willow Project, described by Ketchell and co-workers [14], where the task was to develop a uniform search interface that allows a diverse community of users to retrieve information from heterogeneous, network-based information resources. Willow separates the user interface from the database management or the information retrieval system. It provides a graphic user interface to a variety of information resources residing on diverse hosts. It is based on a "database driver" model, which allows new database hosts to be added without altering Willow itself. Willow employs a multimedia extension mechanism to enable external viewers to handle data in almost any form.

Linking the electronic health record to the digital library is a Web-era reformulation of the long-standing informatics goal of seamless integration of automated clinical data and relevant knowledge-based information to enable informed decisions. The spread of the Internet and the development of the World Wide Web, together with converging format standards for electronic health data and digital publications make effective linking increasingly feasible. Some existing systems link electronic health data and knowledge-based information in limited settings or limited ways. Yet many challenging informatics research problems remain to be solved before flexible and seamless linking becomes a reality and before systems become capable of delivering the specific piece of information needed at the time a decision has to be made [15].

Connecting the electronic health record to the digital library requires positive resolution of important policy issues, including health data privacy, government encouragement of high-speed communications, electronic intellectual property rights, standards for health data and for digital libraries. Both the research problems and the policy issues are items yet to be solved [15].

Shifman et al. developed a case study describing a project that explores issues of quality of service relevant to the next-generation Internet, using the PathMaster application in a test bed environment. PathMaster is a prototype computer system that analyses digitised cell images from cytology specimens and compares the images against an image database, it returns a ranked set of "similar" cell images from the database. To perform next-generation Internet test bed evaluations, a cluster of nine parallel computation workstations were used and configured as three sub-clusters using Cisco routers [16].

At the Vivalog LLC and University of Washington, Seattle an innovative software toolkit was developed that allows the creation of web applications that facilitate the acquisition, integration, and dissemination of multimedia biomedical data over the web. This reduces the cost of knowledge sharing. There is a lack of high-level web application development tools suitable for use by researchers, clinicians, and educators who are not skilled programmers. The Web Interfacing Repository Manager (WIRM) is a software toolkit that reduces the complexity of building customised biomedical web applications. WIRM's visual modelling tools enable domain experts to describe the structure of their knowledge, and WIRM automatically generates full-featured, customisable content management systems [17].

Satellite technology has progressed in the 1990s. The advent of low Earth orbit satellites with their lower power requirements for handheld terminals has allowed rapid advances in telecommunications. Satellite media have been used to provide mobile telemedicine linkages to remote disaster sites as well as military battlefields. In conjunction with this, the development of wireless technologies provided avenues to improve telecommunication capabilities in disasters. Third-generation wireless networks, with unified standards and the ability to provide high-speed, wireless broadband connectivity, are now being explored for multidirectional rapid and real-time audio, video, and other high-density data transmission between users simultaneously. As a result, these new technologies can serve as the basis for a rapid, integrated, wireless communication system for disaster response [18].

The use of information technology (IT) is a key issue for quality health delivery in regional health information networks. Provision of potential technologies for all citizens and health providers in a regional environment, is increasingly emphasised. IT solutions are advanced and continue to evolve user acceptance and friendliness issues are unresolved. Mobile telecommunication solutions may hold the key for wide scale implementation of IT solutions in regional health information networks [19].

A new form of scientific medical meetings has emerged in the last few years — the virtual congress, based on IT technology.

The Internet continues to grow as a delivery medium for health information, and the design of effective Web sites becomes increasingly important. Kinzie provides an overview of one effective model for Web site design. It is a user-centred process that includes techniques for needs assessment, goal/task analysis, user interface design, and rapid prototyping. See <www.healthheritage.net>. This Web site helps patients record and maintain their family health histories in a secure, confidential manner. It also supports physicians through analysis of health histories, identification of potential risks and provision of health care recommendations. Visual examples of the design process are provided to show how the use of this model resulted in an easy-to-use Web site that is likely to meet user needs [20].

2.4 Education and training of the health care staff

Instead of repetitive lectures interactive software should be used. This would increase the efficiency of sub-specialists in teaching institutions. Use of advanced educational designs also could enhance the learning of key features. For many disease states, computer-based instructional multimedia cases are extremely useful teaching tools. This learning format allows the presentation of visual images, sounds, and a wide array of clinical information, enabling the learner to engage in interaction and self-testing, which would improve retention and interest. Typical and atypical visual findings of a disease state can be displayed in a comprehensive manner usually not available in the hit-or-miss outpatient environment. Thus, a certain exposure to informational content can be ensured, freeing the resident-faculty to stress other aspects of patient care. Exposure to telemedicine also should be incorporated into the sub-specialty experience. The speed and efficiency of communication among educators, trainees, and different levels of care providers will also facilitate the educational process modelling generalist. Subspecialist interactions that will become important to paediatric trainees when they move from resident to community practitioner. This modality will become increasingly vital to support generalists in office- or hospital-based practices as they take on more complex roles in care delivery [21].

AI/RHEUM is a multimedia expert system developed originally to assist in the diagnosis of rheumatic diseases in adults. Athreya, Cheh and Kingsland evaluated the usefulness of a modified version of this diagnostic decision support system in diagnosing childhood rheumatic diseases. AI/RHEUM was modified by the addition of 5 new diseases to the knowledge base of the system. Criteria tables for each of the diseases included in the knowledge base were modified to suit the needs of children. The modified system was tested on 94 children seen in a paediatric rheumatology clinic. AI/RHEUM made the correct diagnosis in 92% of the cases when the diagnosis was available in the knowledge base of the system. It was also shown to be effective in the education of paediatric trainees through its multimedia features. During data entry, the physician can use the multimedia capability of the system to obtain expert consultation on each of the patient findings. The multimedia capacity of the program allows for interactive learning and immediate feedback [22].

At the Tokai University Okada, Haruki and Ogushi designed and evaluated a satellite-based Internet system for use in medical applications. Many experimental telemedicine projects use satellites, but they combined digital satellite communication with an ordinary telephone network to realize an economical countrywide network for emergency medicine and continuous medical education. The system appears to be a useful and practical technology for daily clinical activities [23].

Fanaroff recently described some of the challenges facing neonatal medicine: "We must recognize that trainees at all levels learn by doing, not by listening and observing. Medical students, residents and fellows learn better from hands-on experience. Knowledge comes from repeating the experience. It is time to develop multimedia-based interactive training modules that provide really good simulations of possible experiences in a manner similar to the training and recertification of airline pilots." [24] Halamek and co-workers showed that high-fidelity simulation of neonatal resuscitation can be conducted using current technology, that it is well received by those experiencing it for the first time, and that it offers benefits not inherent in traditional medical educational models [25].

Hillenbrand and co-workers describe an interactive multimedia curriculum intervention for paediatric residents to increase their knowledge about common lactation issues. The residents completed questionnaires before and after the intervention to measure knowledge and confidence. Resident behaviours in the clinical setting were measured before and after the intervention using telephone surveys of breastfeeding mothers after a clinic visit with a paediatric resident. These results indicate that not only breastfeeding knowledge and confidence, but most importantly clinical behaviours of paediatric residents can be enhanced through innovative educational opportunities. Appropriate counselling for breastfeeding mothers by paediatricians might contribute to an increase in the duration of breastfeeding [26].

Self-directed and customized medical education programs are gaining importance in health care instruction. In Austria and Germany a repository-driven online computer system (CardioOP) was implemented for teleteaching in Heart Surgery. It supports authoring and multiple re-use of multimedia data for different user groups in different instructional applications and therefore requires a process of content management. Metadata play an important role in the effective discovery and search, access, integration and management of educational multimedia data in medicine. Friedl and co-workers point out at the same time that proper terminology use is also of utmost importance [27].

Learning anatomy and surgical procedures requires both a conceptual understanding of three-dimensional anatomy and a hands-on manipulation of tools and tissue. Such virtual resources are not available widely, are expensive, and may be culturally disallowed. Simulation technology, using high-performance computers and graphics, permits realistic real-time display of anatomy. Haptics technology supports the ability to probe and feel this virtual anatomy through the use of virtual tools. The Internet permits worldwide access to resources. At Stanford University a high-performance server and high-bandwidth communication is used together with Next Generation Internet and complex bimanual haptics to simulate a tool-based learning environment for wide use in the gross anatomy course [28].

Major efforts are being made to improve the teaching of human anatomy to foster cognition of visual-spatial relationships. The Visible Human Project of the National Library of Medicine, as described by Temkin and co-workers, makes it possible to create virtual reality based applications for teaching anatomy. Integration of traditional cadaver and illustration-based methods with Internet-based simulations might bring us closer to this goal [29].

The same authors also dealt with the Web-based three-dimensional Virtual Body Structures (W3D-VBS). This is a next-generation, immersive, anatomical training system for teaching human anatomy over the Internet. It uses visible human data to dynamically explore, select, extract, visualize, manipulate, and stereoscopically palpate realistic virtual body structures with a haptic device. Tracking the user's progress through evaluation tools helps customize lesson plans. A self-guided "virtual tour" of the whole body allows investigation of labelled virtual dissections repetitively, at any time and place a user requires it [29].

2.5 Standards

Just as important as the above questions are the questions of standards and quality.

Tirado-Ramos, Hu, and Lee asserted that representations of the DICOM (Digital Imaging and Communications for Medicine) Structured Reporting standard, using object-oriented modelling languages such as the Unified Modelling Language, can provide a high-level reference view of the semantically rich framework of DICOM and its complex structures. They have produced an object-oriented model to represent the DICOM SR standard and have derived XML-exchangeable representations of this model using World Wide Web Consortium specifications [30].

Many people know of Health Level 7 (HL7) as an organization that creates health care messaging standards. Health Level 7 is also developing standards for the representation of clinical documents (such as discharge summaries and progress notes). These document standards make up the HL7 Clinical Document Architecture (CDA). The HL7 CDA Framework, release 1.0, became an ANSI-approved HL7 standard in November 2000. The CDA is a document mark-up standard that specifies the structure and semantics of clinical documents. A CDA document is a defined and complete information object that can include text, images, sounds, and other multimedia content [31].

2.6 The education of the patients

An automated computer interview would be an interesting approach to introducing IT in the field of patient – computer interaction. Lenert and Soetikno experimented with such a system, and developed a program to train subjects in the use of different preference assessment methods, presented descriptions of mild post-thrombotic syndrome (PTS), severe PTS and stroke and elicited subject preferences for these health states. They developed a computerized instrument to measure preferences in 30 community volunteers and 30 internal medicine physicians, to elicit patient preferences. Their method appeared to be a practical and valid approach to individualizing therapy [32].

Tetzlaff described a questionnaire system to help evoke a picture of home care informatics needs: The questionnaire was used to evaluate information needs and assess programmable technologies. It was distributed to a clinical population of parents of children with cancer. On-line systems can offer breadth, depth and timeliness currently unattainable. Multimedia solutions appear to complement user needs and preferences. Patients should be involved in the formation and development process in much the same way that users are involved in user centred computer interface design [33].

At the University of Wisconsin-Milwaukee already in 1998 a project called "The Layman Education and Activation System" was introduced. It aimed to prepare people to take a more active role in their health care decisions. It was designed to be an interactive, Internet-based system for collecting the patient's medical history. It gave patients access to educational information when this was most pertinent, while they were attempting to complete a form. It avoided overwhelming the patient, by providing information only when it was likely to be relevant. The system tailored the content of the form to the patient's responses. The system also used the patient's answers to suggest questions that the patient might ask a doctor and provided online resources that the patient could browse [34].

Homer and co-workers described an interactive multimedia asthma education computer program that provided patients with the substantive knowledge required for good asthma care and supplied a simulated environment in which children and their families could safely gain experience with asthma-related contingent decision-making. Educational theory supported linking the teaching of a desired set of actions, such as asthma management, with a desirable pastime activity for children, such as playing video/computer games [35].

In another study two hundred and twenty-eight children with asthma visiting a paediatric pulmonary clinic were randomly assigned to control and intervention groups. Children and caregivers in both groups received traditional patient education based on the National Asthma Education and Prevention Program. Intervention group participants received additional self-management education through the Interactive Multimedia Program for Asthma Control and Tracking. Pediatric Asthma Care Knowledge Survey, Pediatric Asthma Caregiver's Quality of Life Questionnaire. Asthma symptom history, spirometry, and health services utilization data were collected at the initial visit and at 3 and 12 months. Supplementing conventional asthma care with interactive multimedia education has significantly improved asthma knowledge and reduced the burden of childhood asthma [36].

Shegog and co-workers described a prospective pre-test and post-test randomised intervention trial to assess the motivational appeal of a computer-assisted instructional program and evaluated the impact of the program in eliciting change in knowledge, self-efficacy, and attributions of children with asthma. Subjects were recruited from large urban asthma clinics, community clinics, and schools. Seventy-six children 9 to 13 years old were recruited for the evaluation. Their program, called "Watch, Discover, Think and Act", was an intrinsically motivating educational program that had the ability to effect determinants of asthma self-management behaviour in 9- to 13-year-old children with asthma. This, coupled with its reported effectiveness in enhancing patient outcomes in clinical settings, indicated that this program has an application in paediatric asthma education [37].

Focus group discussions and individual interviews were conducted in five European countries to ascertain the needs of caregivers in this area, as described by Chambers and co-workers. The findings were used to design a three-part multimedia software application to help family caregivers prepare to cope with sudden, unexpected, and difficult situations that might arise during their time as a caregiver. This prototype then was evaluated via user trials and usability questionnaires to consider the usability and acceptance of the application. User acceptance of the software application was high, and the key features of usability such as content, appearance, and navigation were highly rated. In general, comments were positive and enthusiastic regarding the content of the software application and relevance to the caring situation. The software application had the potential to offer information and support to those who are caring for the elderly and disabled at home and to help them prepare for a crisis [38].

An aim of the program developed by Fenney and co-workers was to develop and evaluate the effectiveness of a CD-ROM–based multimedia program as a tool to increase user's knowledge of the differences between "normal" forgetfulness and more serious memory loss associated with Alzheimer's disease. The program was most effective for participants with a lower level of self-reported prior knowledge about memory loss and Alzheimer's disease. Viewers particularly valued having personal access to a confidential source that permitted them to become informed about memory loss without public disclosure. This multimedia CD-ROM technology program provided an efficient and effective means of teaching older adults about memory loss and ways to distinguish benign from serious memory loss. It uniquely balanced public community outreach education and personal privacy [39].

An Internet-based telemedicine program designed to reduce the costs of care and to provide enhanced medical, informational, and emotional support to families who have infants with very low birth weight during and after their neonatal intensive care unit stay, was evaluated by Gray and co-workers: Baby CareLink is a multifaceted telemedicine program that incorporates videoconferencing and World Wide Web (WWW) technologies to enhance interactions between families, staff, and community providers. The videoconferencing module allows virtual visits and distance learning from a family's home during an infant's hospitalisation as well as virtual house calls and remote monitoring after discharge. Baby CareLink's WWW site contains information on issues that confront these families. In addition, its security architecture allows efficient and confidential sharing of patient-based data and communications among authorized hospital and community users [40].

The key to managing food allergies in schools successfully is to train the staff to minimize risks, recognize symptoms, and act quickly once a reaction occurs. The FAAN's School Food Allergy Program is a multimedia comprehensive program designed to aid the school staff in developing a school-wide food allergy awareness program. The 'Be A PAL: Protect A Life From Food Allergies' program educates classmates about how they can help prevent a reaction. Both of these programs have been well-received and are in place in thousands of school across the United States [41].

Patient-centred information management may overcome barriers that impede high-quality, safe care in the emergency department. The utility of parents' report of medication data via a multimedia, touch screen interface, the asthma kiosk, was investigated by Porter et al. Their specific aims were to estimate the validity of parents' electronically entered medication history for asthma and to compare the parents' kiosk entries regarding medications to the documentation of emergency department physicians and nurses [42].

2.7 Patients rehabilitation programs

An important task is also the proper education of and helps for the patients themselves. Multimedia programs can be of assistance to the patients by providing information, giving them therapy sometimes in the form of entertainment (important for children) and helping them in their everyday chores.

Computer play can provide good support for children who have not previously been able to play in a "meaningful" way. Many parents of children with profound intellectual impairments and multiple disabilities complain that they experience difficulties in stimulating their child and state that he/she does not play independently and that is very passive. Parents thus require advice and help on how to play and stimulate a child with profound disabilities. A new way to stimulate and engage a child may be to use computers. Parents often have high expectation of computers as tools for play, probably based on applications used in other fields of the information society [43].

In the next sections we will cover specifically questions related to low vision, hearing and motor- impaired patients.

2.7.1 Programs for low vision patients

In the early 1980's computers become more available for visually impaired children in schools [44] and a significant number of software systems were developed to support the assessment and training of visual skills [45, 46]. Recently systems have been produced for the more modern computer systems available today. These systems can be used to support a subset of visual skills, namely: awareness of vision as a sense, localization of visual stimuli, colour vision, tracking and hand-eye co-ordination [47].

In order to support computer use among children and young people with disabilities, a pilot project with eight computer play centres was started in Sweden some years ago. Parents and children with disabilities were invited to visit a computer play centre without a referral from a medical doctor. The staffs working at the centres were well-educated and had a wide knowledge of children with disabilities as they previously worked at the child development centres. They were a mixture of special educators, occupational therapists, speech therapists and sometimes technicians. They worked as a team and their job was to assist families of children with disabilities to find suitable software, make adaptations of the hardware (computer and keyboard) and give parents and children advice about play and child development [48].

Over the past two decades, the blind and the visually impaired have been experiencing striking improvements in their access to information: These improvements have come about through the general trend in society to store and distribute information in digital form and by introducing a technology that makes the computer accessible to the blind. By replacing the computer screen with a refreshable Braille display or a speech synthesizer, files stored on a computer can be accessed, and software operated by a blind individual. Optical character recognition and speech synthesizer software open the world of printed material to the blind reader. Unfortunately, these very advantageous trends are confined to textual information, whereas graphic materials are still almost inaccessible [49].

The Tactile Interactive Multimedia (TIM) project, described by Archambault et al [50] is a project whose main objective was to offer to visually impaired children of various levels of psychomotor development the possibility to play computer games in an autonomous way. TIM included high level research on cognitive psychology and education sciences in order to ensure a high level of quality allowing blind children in early youth to use a computer, like sighted children. The software gives the computer a double role: entertainment and educational. For some children, having additional disabilities, e.g. cognitive difficulties, it can have a third role as a therapeutic tool [51]. A game platform, the blindstation, was developed to adapt existing content or create new games. It provides a set of Python functions to describe those games in an abstract way, independently from their representation. The platform can then deliver the game in a multi-modal way using the screen, keyboard or a speech synthesizer. The delivery is selected either dependent on the available devices or on the user's choices and disabilities [52].

Many children who have damage to the temporal or occipital lobe of the brain suffer from visual perception disorders (VPD). Persons suffering from visual agnosias, agnosias of colour, size discrimination disorders, prosopagnosia and hemineglecton of visual fields were rehabilitated in the past by using various training aids such as colour cards, drawn geometrical figures, objects, letters, painted pictures etc. The aim of work of Ruseckaite and Lukauskiene was to evaluate new methods for the rehabilitation of VPD by using some form of computerized program. They trained and rehabilitated with various kinds of VPD and were able to develop new skills from the results of intensive training. They tested over 450 children with damaged right and left temporal lobes of brain. They used the Munsel colour recognition test. The method could be used to restore some kinds of visual agnosia in children with damaged hemispheres of brain [53].

Some designers develop not only for visually impaired children but for blind children too. The European Media Master of Arts program of the Utrecht School of the Arts (Arts, Media and Technology) and the Bartiméus Accessibility Foundation in Zeist have developed a curriculum for program development. Within this curriculum many spectacular games have been developed already like Drive, The Curb Game, Hall of Sound, Powerchors, Wow, Demor and others. Panels have been developed from the users of these games to investigate the future direction of gaming [54].

The number of partially sighted children increases year to year. Several games of different types (action, adventure, exploration…) have already been developed for them. There are also many instruments for partially sighted people [55], including some very new solutions [56], but not for very small children.

2.7.2 Programs for hearing impaired patients

In general, it is difficult to establish communication between the visually and the hearing impaired. At the Tsukuba College of Technology a chat application was developed that has user interfaces for both the visually and the hearing impaired. Access to the program had the highest priority for visually impaired. To discover how to realize a natural communication on the network for hearing impaired was difficult [57]. A "Chatting System" was developed based on an Internet Relay Chat to create communication between visually and hearing impaired students. The developed software creates speech using a screen reader program for the visually impaired users. By means of this system, these impaired students could communicate through the Internet in real time even if they were far apart from each other [58].

The Lipcom project is a research and development effort by IBM France; it seeks to assist spoken communication from hearing to deaf persons, by providing a full phonetic transcription of speech in real time, which, when combined with other sources of information (lip movements, hearing aid, etc), would assist in the perception of speech [59].

SIMOLE (Multimedia System for Reading Comprehension Instruction) is a computer program to train reading comprehension skills in adult deaf people. It is basically a self-learning application [60].

2.7.3 Programs for children with moving and multiple handicapped

Pimlott, Blenkhorn and Evans made a prototype adaptation to a standard Graphical User Interface that was designed to allow a person with a physical disability to interact more easily with the operating system and software applications [61].

In a Spanish project an alternative browsing interface was developed for people with severe motor impairment who work with scanning selections sets to browse the web [62].

The needs of those users whose severe motor impairments force them to use exclusively a switch controlled scanning system to work with the computer cannot be properly addressed today. To find the best access system depends very much on the user. But the programming option is very expensive in terms of development cost, especially when we consider that the present evolution of Internet could make obsolete any browsing application in only a couple of years [63].

A technical assistance system has been developed by the Vienna University of Technology. The main focus has been to provide new means to support the development of severely and multiply disabled children giving them more independence and autonomy while exploring their material and social environment [64].

2.7.4 Program for aphasic patients

While the cost of therapists could be eased by virtual self-help groups in geographical areas but many people suffering from aphasia are not able to interact with current chat tools. This is because massive word finding difficulties can lead to typing a simple sentence taking up to several minutes. Spaniol, Springer Klamma and Jarke designed and implemented and evaluated new chat tool for such groups [65].

3. The Multimedia Programs Developed at The University of Veszprém

At the University of Veszprém our group started the development of educational multimedia programs for special needs users some ten years ago. Since then a great deal of such software has been completed. Recently the interest of our group has been directed towards developing virtual reality programs, especially with the needs of disabled people in mind. In this section we will provide an overview of our programs.

3.1 The 'Tale landscape" program for low vision children

Of particular importance was the design of the main menu of our program [66] called Tale landscape. It had to provide a well-organized screen layout while not interfering with the mood of the story. The main menu is a picture of a landscape from bird's-eye view, where different parts of the landscape correspond to different menu items, and every item provides a separate game (see Figure 1). If the mouse is placed over such an object of the screen, a frame shows that it is a valid selection.

In this program the tasks are games:

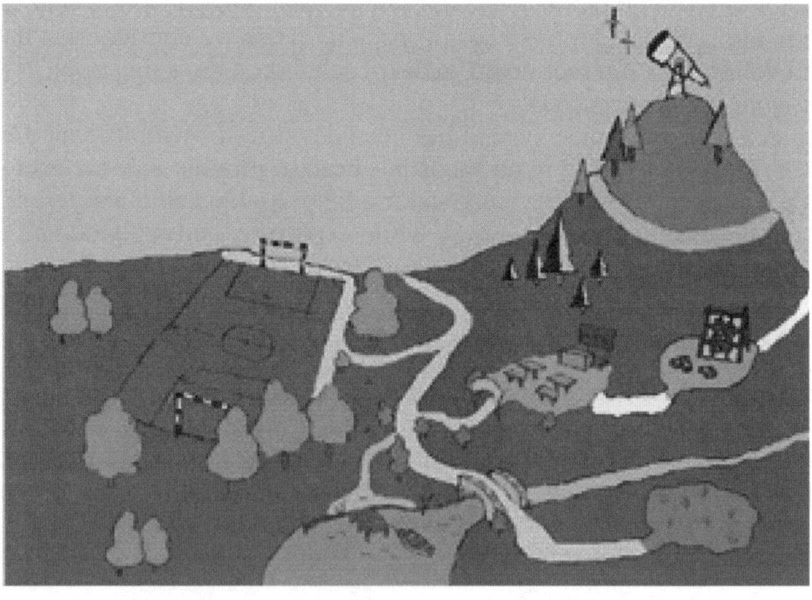

Fig. 1. The main menu of "Tale landscape" multimedia software.

'Find the opening!"game

In this game a Landolt ring test can be conducted. The Landolt ring looks like a letter C. The task is to determine from different distances the opening direction of the Landolt-ring, which is rotated by the program. The user (teacher) can set the parameters: the size of the ring, its colour and texture, the colour of the background. The test can also run using the capital letter E instead of a Landolt ring. In this case one has to determine the direction of the fork openings.

'Black and white"game

In this task the screen is divided into two parts. On the left side different objects can be seen, on the right side the inverses of the same objects. The task is to find the corresponding objects on the two sides.

'Catch it!"game

In this simple game the task is to catch one of the moving animals with the net.

'Recognize it!"game

This game has two versions. The first is the easier task. On the display the picture of an animal appears, and the child has to tell what he/she has seen. The pictures change at random. The picture disappears after a given time, and then one has to guess what one had seen, or one can make a new trial.

The second version is a more difficult form of this game. As can be seen in Figure 2 three objects are displayed simultaneously. They each have to be recognized.

'Small differences"game

This is a computer variation of the well-known task to observe small differences. Figure 3 shows an example. The two pictures differ only in some slight details. One has to click with the mouse on to the differences observed. The little raindrops in the upper right corner show how many differences have to be found.

'Puzzle"game

In this game the picture has been subdivided into 3 x 3 rectangles. With the help of the mouse the location of two rectangles can be changed. The child has to re-create the original picture.

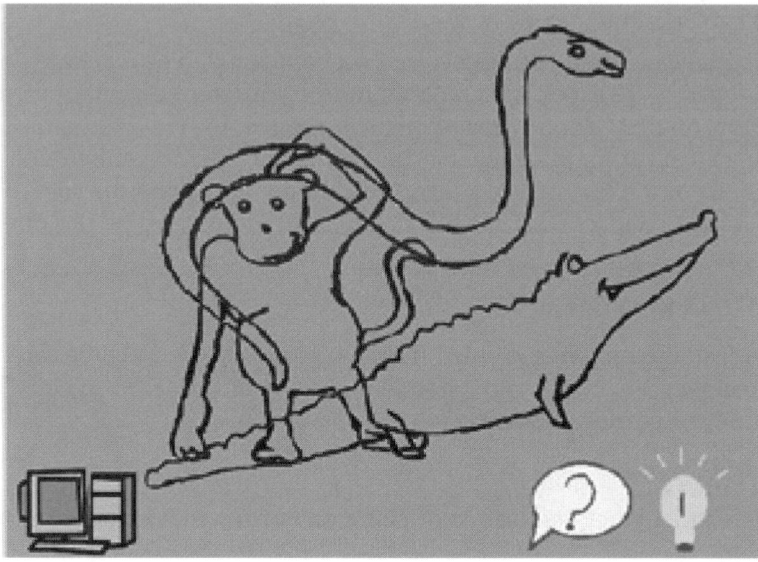

Fig. 2. Recognize it game

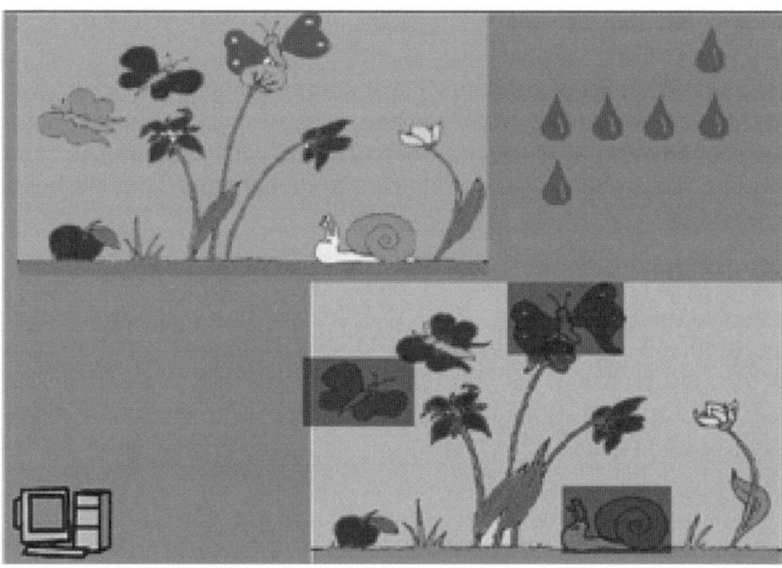

Fig. 3. Small differences game

'Star''game

A further game is the Star-game. Here the single stars have to be connected by a line to become the outlined of a familiar object. Compared to similar paper and pencil tasks the difference is that much more complicated arrangements of the stars can be used, because the star that is the next in the sequence changes its size periodically and the child has to see this movement.

'Football"game

One has to move the ball with the help of the mouse and get it into the goal. But one has to be careful not to hit the goalkeeper (the hedgehog). One can set the size of the ball, to make it easier to see. This however makes it more difficult to aim.

3.2 Evaluation of the 'Tale landscape"Program for low vision children

To evaluate the usefulness of our programs, we designed a questionnaire and sent it to special schools together with the programs, asking them to test the programs and give their opinion on their usefulness by filling in the attached questionnaire.

So far eight groups have tested the programs and have sent back the filled in questionnaire. We have asked eight questions on the acceptance and usefulness of the programs, and requested to opinion of the teachers using a five-step scale, where 1 was the lowest mark, and 5 the best. The questions, the average mark the teachers gave, together with the standard deviation of the marks is reproduced in Table 1.

Table 1: Evaluation of the feedback received from different groups.

Question	Average mark	Standard deviation
How well does the program help to ameliorate the visus of the children?	4.0	0.8
How well do the training and the games suit the children?	4.0	0.8
Is the wording understandable to the children?	4.4	0.5
Does the program motivate the children?	3.9	0.8
Are the pictures appealing to the children?	3.5	0.8
Is the tutorial character of the program adequate?	3.6	0.5
Does the use of the program attract the children?	3.7	0.8
Is the navigation system and the interactivity of the programs adequate.	3.8	0.5

As can be seen from this table the acceptance of the programs was very good and the children liked to use them (Question 1 and 2). This is most important for training their eyes.

The general comment was that the children enjoyed "playing" with the programs, thus they perceived the tasks they had to execute as a game, not a burden. As mentioned the most important outcome from the use of the new medium to train the lazy eye of the child (in case of ambyopia). In the questionnaire we have not asked about other issues that were obvious: that the computer version avoids the wastage of paper cards, its easy re-use, and its adaptability to the level of the lazyness of the eye (line width, contrast of the pictures, etc.).

The advantages range from the higher motivation of the child to the adaptability to the individual requirements of the patient.

3.3 Programs for hearing impaired children

The first program is "Now I know already what its name is" [67]. The main menu has eight topics. For example School, Christmas, Easter, Garden, Summer, In the hospital and so on (Fig. 4).

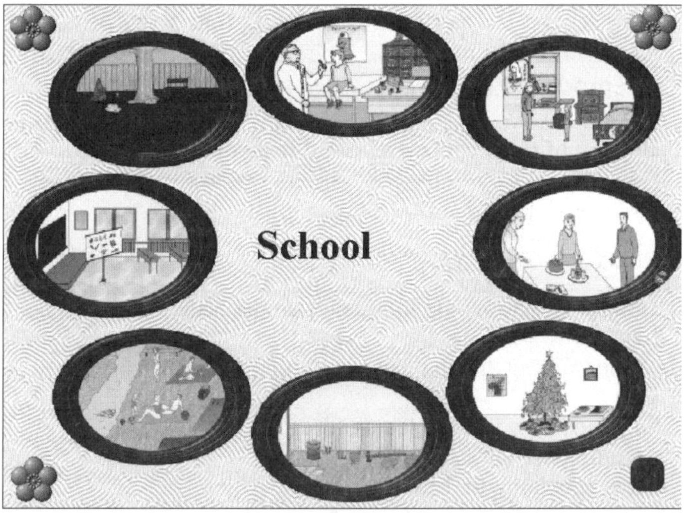

Fig. 4. The main menu of the first program with the mouse pointing to the school sub menu.

If you click on a picture, you can go into a sub menu. In the sub menu of a topic there are two other sub menus. The painting and the talking sub menus (Fig. 5). Every talking submenu has a cartoon like presentation, because we saw, when we were in the special school for deaf children that they like cartoons. Why? Because they have a lot of pictures and not less text.

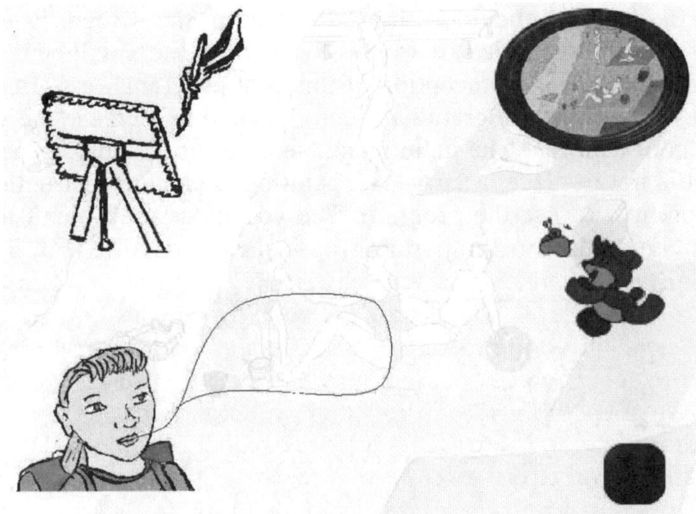

Fig. 5. One of the sub menus of the first program

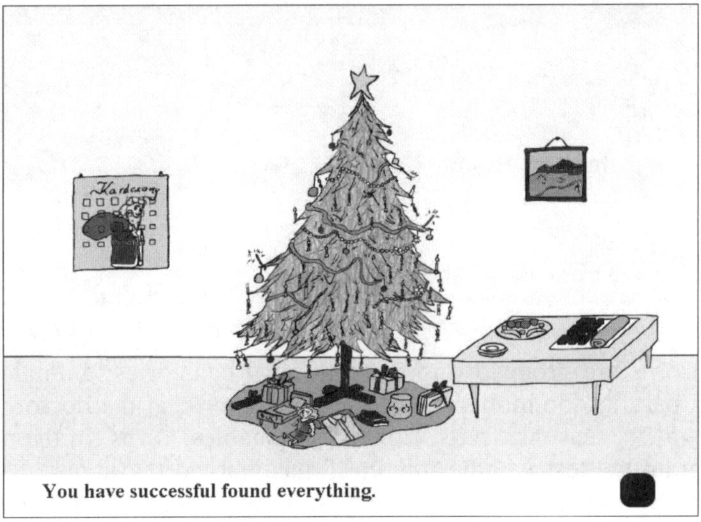

Fig. 6. One figure from the painting submenu

The painting sub menu is the real task for the children. The picture shows a scene where objects are shown only in black and white. The program asks a question, written below the picture. For example – Where is the cake? (Fig. 6) If the child clicks on the right place in the screen, it will be coloured. If she or he can identify every object, all of them will be coloured.

Based on the positive reception of this first program we started a second one [67]. The second program has been prepared to increase the vocabulary of the school children. The main menu has five sub-menus: vocabulary, one item that is not in place, a fairy-tale, painting, and short instructions for the teacher on how to use the program. The vocabulary sub-menu has 14 sections containing the most important words of everyday life (Fig. 7).

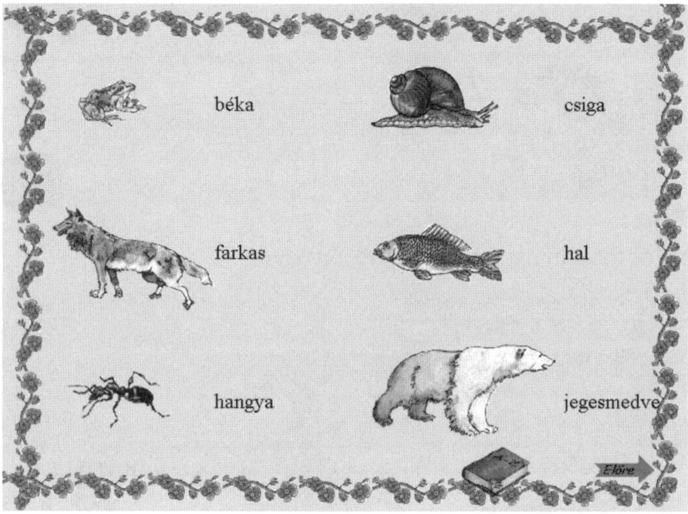

Fig. 7. One page from the vocabulary submenu

The words are grouped into the following categories: animals, domestic animals, parts of the human body, clothing, sports, at the doctor, the house, school, traffic, seasons, fruits, flowers, vegetables, verbs. In the next part of the program we test whether the child has learned the name of the objects correctly: Several objects are shown, and the sentence at the bottom of the page asks the child to identify one item in the picture (Fig. 8).

The child has to point to the item with the mouse. Deaf children might have difficulty with this identification. In addition there are tales and colouring submenus. In the tale submenu there are well known tales. The tale is depicted in 4 to 5 slides, with the tale itself written at the bottom of the slide, and above the text there is a picture showing an episode from the tale.

In the colouring submenu an episode becomes visible. Below the picture there is a question, e.g. asking the child to point to an object in the picture. If the child points with the cursor to the correct object the black and white part of the picture turns into colour, and a new question is seen under the picture.

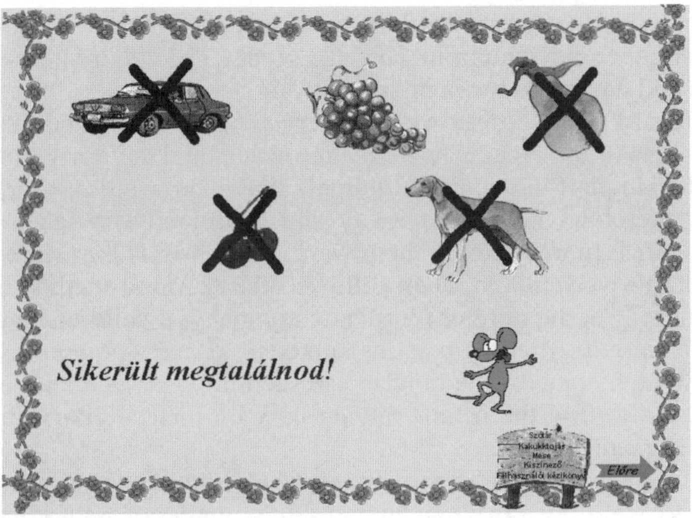

Fig. 8. One item that is not in place submenu

3.4 Efficiency test of the multimedia program for hearing impaired children

The efficiency tests of both software systems were performed in the Török Béla Kindergarten, Elementary School and Special Trade School in Budapest. The students of this school have various type and intensity of hearing difficulties. This test was carried out with children in the age group of 5-7 years. These children had normal mental ability. It would be interesting to test the software with children who have learning difficulties too.

Both types of software were very popular in the 5-7 years age group. They were used in the individual and group training of the mother-tongue language classes. Both types of software develop primarily active and passive vocabulary. But they also offer several more possibilities. They can be used for the development of reading and hearing skills. These together help the learning of speech.

The advantages of the software are the easy navigation and simple tasks. The children understood the tasks very quickly. They worked together in pairs, but they could also work individually. Learning the use of the next and the back button was very easy so the children were highly motivated. The first attempt is very important for every child and immediate success provides positive feedback.

The topics of the first "Now I know its name" software suits the mother-tongue language curriculum for this age group. The children easily selected the tasks and navigated the main menu well.

With regard to the figures we used very simple pictures, because the previous designs of the pictures were overcrowded, and the navigation was difficult. The simple figures, like children's drawings, were reassuring for the children; therefore they could easily and confidently navigate within the simple figures. In every topic there were 3 or 4 words that were not yet in the children's vocabulary. They followed the learning method accurately, and in this way at the third or fourth attempt many of children could find the objects requested. After the painting submenu, if every object was coloured, and the written name of the objects vanished, the task was for ear-training, i.e. they had to find the details relying only on their auditory channel, excluding lip-reading.

After that there was speech training, the children had to recite the names of the objects. In this development period the main goal was correct articulation.

The topics the children especially enjoyed were: the school, the beach, Christmas and at the doctors.

The second software offered different possibilities for the expansion of vocabulary, explanation of words, their auditory differentiation and training based on hearing. Children could easily navigate in the menu. Finding the odd words was only difficult for children with severe impairments, but it provided them with further new knowledge. The reward of the animations was very popular; the success was so great, that the children in most cases jumped in front of the mirror and imitated the movement and dancing of the animals. The dancing animals were the reward.

3.5 For motor-impaired children

We prepared two programs [68] for physically disabled children (Pedagogical test similar to the S.O.N. test and a memory toy). The programs are designed for disabled children, thus they have to be user friendly and easy to use. The children can work with the traditional keyboard, with the help of Intellikeys, or with the mouse, or with a switch if they cannot use the mouse. In this case the child waits for the movement of a little blue rectangle in the SON test and the memory toy.

SON test: The pedagogical investigation part of the program is based on the idea of the SON (Snijders – Oomen) test. It is a non-verbal intelligence test. The program contains several tasks the child will experience as a game. This test has no time limit.

The tasks are grouped around a main program called "story-tree" (Fig. 9). Parts of it are: Pictures that belong together, analogies, sorting tasks, combinations, memory tasks, filling in, and ordering pictures.

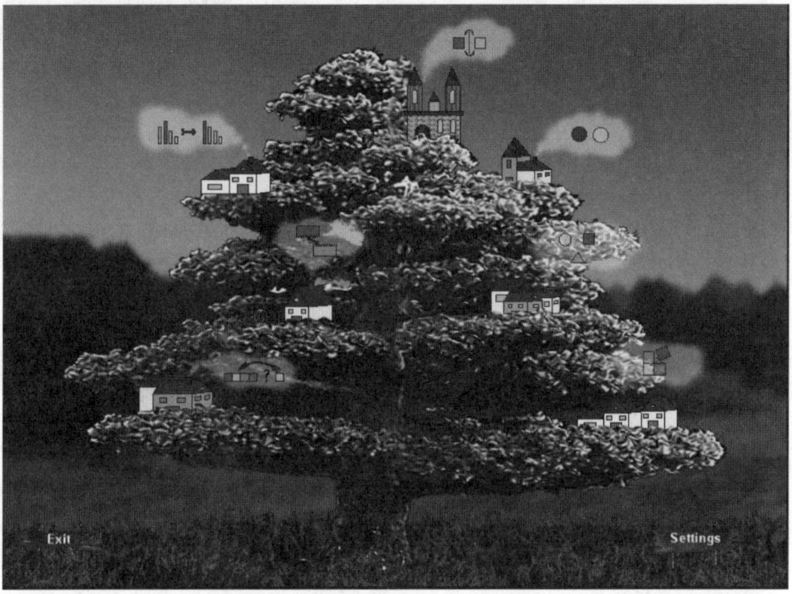

Fig. 9. The main program called "story-tree".

After selecting the task type we get into a room, where we can select to move to the task a or b. There is a small picture of the story-tree on the wall; this signals that we can get back into the main menu by clicking it (Fig. 10).

Memory pictures: On the lower part of the monitor screen there are three hidden pictures, on the upper part there are six hidden pictures. In this task only one picture can be seen at a time. First one of the pictures appears in the lower row.

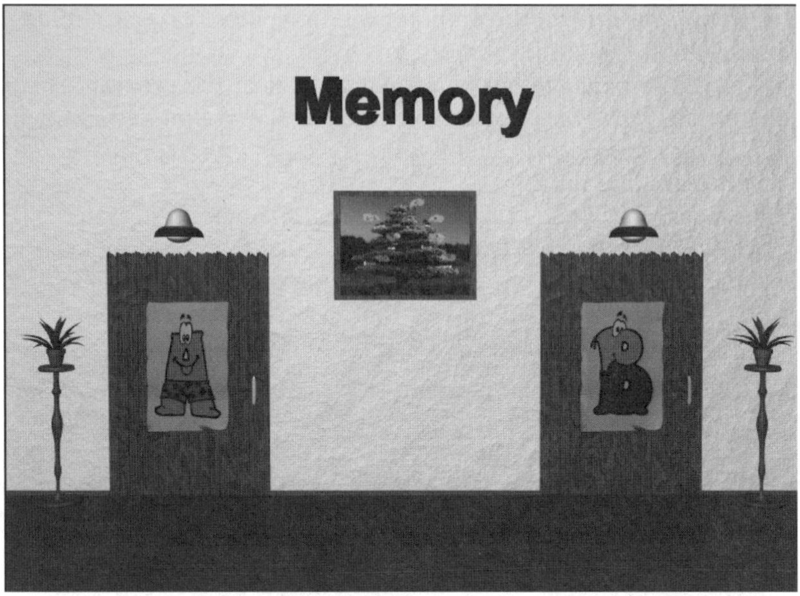

Fig. 10. The sub menu

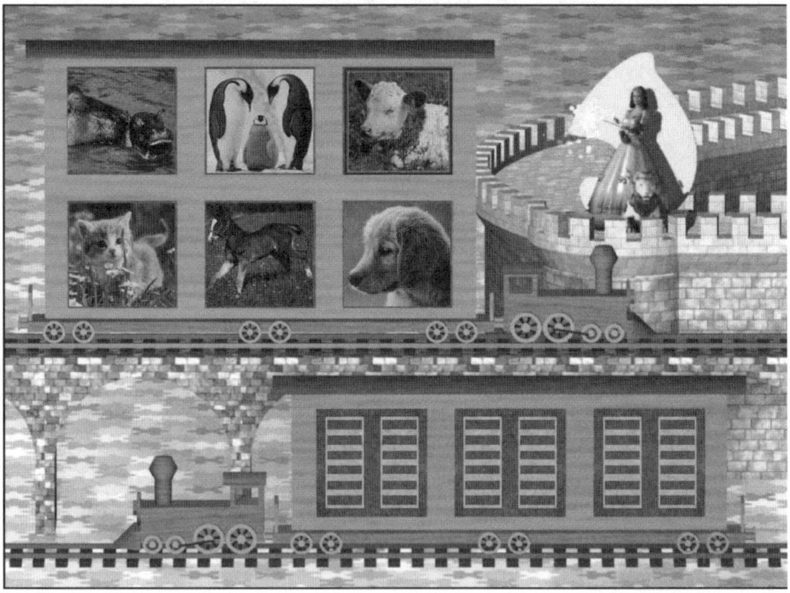

Fig. 11. Memory-pictures task

Then all pictures appear in the upper train. The child must find the corresponding picture here to the picture it has seen for a short time in the lower part of the screen. If the answer is correct answer, as seen in the slide, the child gets a reward from the fairy (Fig. 11).

Relationships-I: Here a cyclic raw is produced on the screen, similar to the work sheets used in kindergartens, and this sequence has to be continued. Thus e.g. green rod, white rod, green rod, white rod, green rod etc., or red circle, red circle, blue circle, red circle, red circle, blue circle, continue. You can imagine that such a task would be hard without a computer for somebody who has motor difficulties

Relationship-II: The task is to find the pair of figures. Every picture in the lower train has a pair in the upper train.

Combination: In this task the child builds a picture from the three part pictures in the lower train. It is a hard task too.

In the memory (Fig. 12) toy one has to match pictures, for example, number of points to the number, lines to figures, capital letters to capital letters, small letters to small letters, the first character of a word to a picture, the second character of a word to a picture, the third character of a word to a picture. This part of the program also contains a toy using logical work sheets. In this part we have re-designed conventional work sheets in a computerised form. The animated or jumping number and animated character in the 4th row were the children's favourite memory toys (Fig. 13).

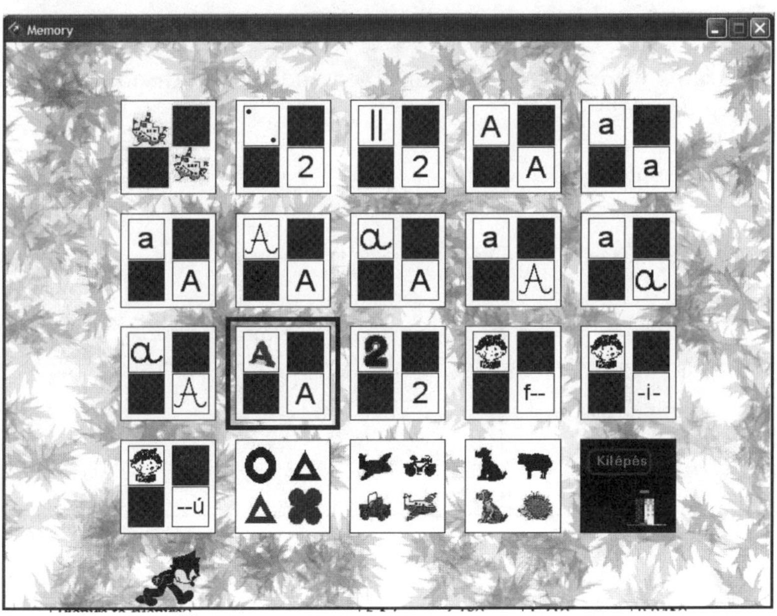

Fig. 12. The main menu of the Memory toy

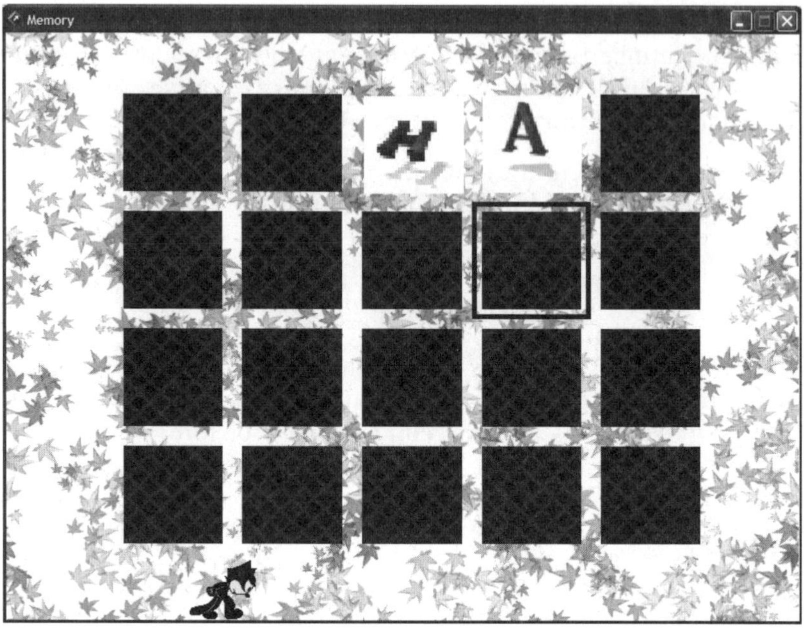

Fig. 13. Jumping letters

3.6. Pedagogical test of the software

The programs were tested by 20 disabled and 20 non-disabled children. The results are the following:

Table 2: The result of SON test

The result of SON test	Disabled	Non-disabled	Level of significance
	Average error	Average error	
Memory of 1 picture	0,5	0	0,075
Memory of 5 pictures	3,33	2	0,047
Analogies (row)	1,7	0,93	0,002
Analogies (figure)	1,73	2	0,028
Combination	1,4	1	0,026

Table 3: The results of the Memory toy

Memory toy	Disabled		Non-disabled	Level of significance
	Time (sec)		Time (sec)	
Picture to picture	6,52	3,18	1,21	0,045
First character to pictures	8	6,04	1,56	0,003
Second character to picture	9,02	7,51	2,35	<0.001
Jumping number to standing number	3,12	1,49	1,06	<0.001
Jumping character to standing character	3,55	2,25	1,34	<0.001

In the second column of Table 3 the first number shows the results with the moving blue rectangles, the second number shows the result with mouse clicking. To calculate the level of significance only the mouse clicking results were used. There are significant differences among the groups. The reason is that the disabled children are slow, because they cannot use the mouse or keyboard as non-disabled children can and they must wait for the moving blue rectangle. Another reason is that although these children were of the same age group as the children of the control group they were studying in a lower class. They are 2 classes behind be-cause they have to first attend preparatory classes. In Hungary the mathe- matics teaching is good, but hard. The non-disabled children have a lot of mathematics experience in those two years, therefore they had better results. We are convinced that the disabled children with motor difficulties are as bright as the control group.

3.7 Program for stroke patients

The "HELEN" cognitive diagnostics and rehabilitation method is a computer controlled method (HELp Neuropsychology = HELEN) which enables – in contrast to methods used internationally – not only the establishment of the diagnosis, but permits measurement of the effectiveness of the therapy [69].

The system we have developed provides help for neuropsychological clinicians by supporting them in setting up the anamnesis, providing tests and training material for rehabilitation work and keeping track of patients' progress.

The system contains a form for holding patients' personal data, numerous tests and tutorial tasks, and a database in which the rehabilitation process is archived. The single tasks contain decision-making situations, and the system provides assistance when the patient seeks it. In case of failure the system provides the possibility of a new trial. The method used by the patient to solve the problems is stored, as this represents important information for the neurologist. To enable the patient to find his or her best solution to the problem, we have developed interactive procedures that permit the solution to be reached using different cognitive approaches. It was important that the different routes taken by patients should not influence the test results, which are expressed in points, but should guide the rehabilitation process.

During the diagnostic phase of the rehabilitation, the program keeps track of the patient's problem-solving strategy and uses this to select the best rehabilitation plan. In order to do this, we use syndrome analysis, thus our system is not merely a collection of computerized tests, but has been built in such a way that it uses the solution provided by the patient to select the next task. The system contains tasks that relate to perception, memory and attention, including writing, reading and counting tasks. In addition, a new aspect of our solution is that, through modern technical support, the difficulty of the task can be changed by using colouring, changing the local or global stroke intensity, or adding noise.

The program also presents numerically the efficiency of the task solution. This means that diagnostic and therapeutic programs are not only used according to the individual needs, but also supply exact results and comparative data. One can therefore investigate cognitive and behaviour deficits in such a way as to activate the intact functions of the brain, thereby allowing the patient to control the course of the procedures. The pace of the rehabilitation is thus influenced by the cooperation of the patient, and by this involvement it is hoped that the speed of rehabilitation will also increase. In addition, the main menu of the HELEN program is constructed to allow new tests and practice tasks to be added at any time.

3.8 The specification of the logical structure of the HELEN software

The following data are stored in the database of the software:

- personal data
- left- or right-handedness (this has to be known to ensure the best strategy for certain tasks)
- data from the investigation, e.g. test results stored in the different submenus of the program, their solution strategy, drawings prepared by the patient, audio recordings, etc.

The HELEN system contains several interactive computer-controlled rehabilitation programs. Using these programs the neurologist can reveal individual changes in the mental capacity of the patient, and can get new information on the cognitive functioning of the patient's brain. The program can be used also in group therapies.

The tasks of the HELEN interactive and therapeutic test and teaching software:

a. Tasks to be used via the Internet

- How many pictures do you see?
- How many black and white chequered drawings do you see?
- How many black and white chequered drawings do you see?
- Where?
- Memory game
- Concealed pictures
- Concealed pictures

b. Therapeutic tests

- Picture with noisy background
- Stories similar to the Binet pictures
- Ordering according to form and colour
- Recognition of emotions
- Identify!
- Ordering of pictures
- Recognition of faces
- Ordering of sentences
- Logical cards
- Clock
- Blind map
- Story

During the task the patient can ask for help if he/she feels he/she needs it. In the tasks of our system the difficulty of the task can be changed using colouring, changing the local or global intensity or by adding noise.

3.8.1 Some tasks in detail:

Puzzle:

To begin with we can see the pieces of a jig saw picture dispersed and rotated at the border of the screen. On the border of the picture we can see the outlines of the piece to be inserted. The picture is fit into a frame. The program saves:

- The order of the chosen pieces (It's important to know whether the patient is left or right handed, because he or will have different starting points)
- If the patient tries to put a piece in the wrong place
- If he or she gives up inserting the chosen piece and chooses a new one
- the help given

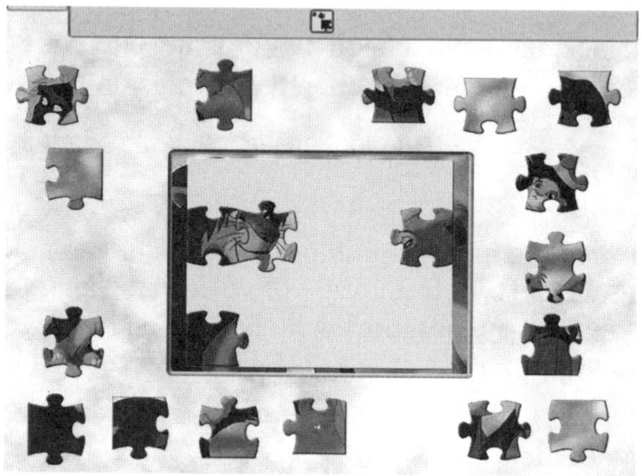

Fig. 14. Puzzle

How many pictures do you see?

On the screen 2D figures can be seen drawn on top of each other. The task is to identify the number of the figures. The program can help by colouring the figures, or it chooses one and shades it (Fig. 15). The program saves the attempts and the help given.

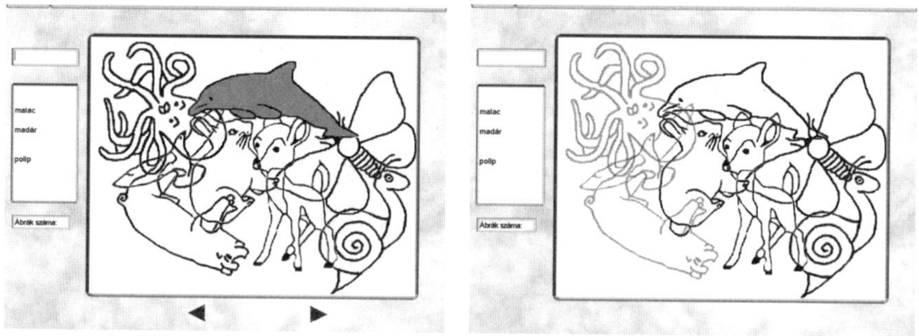

Fig. 15. How many pictures do you see?

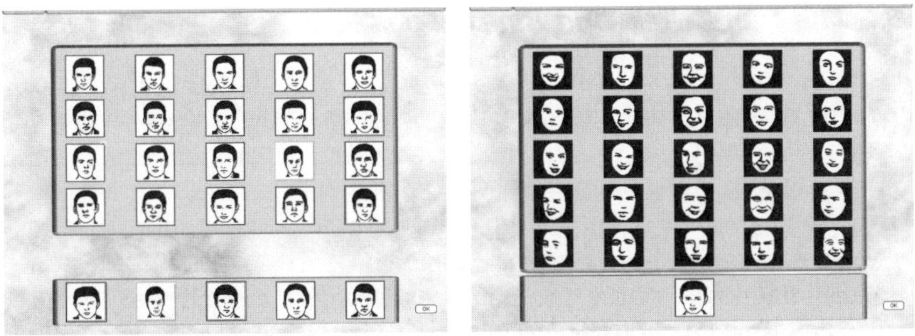

Fig. 16. Recognition of faces

Recognition of faces

20 black and white faces can be seen on the screen. The patient sees 5 of them at the bottom of the screen. His task is to find the matching ones (Fig 16).

At the next step he/she can see 25 faces showing emotion for 10 seconds. When they disappear a face from the first set can be seen on the screen. The patient can memorize the face for as long as he/she wants. When he/she hits a key, he/she has to choose the face from the first set of 20 faces (Fig 16).

Recognition of emotions

16 pictures of emotions of the same woman can be seen (indifferent, happy, amazed, angry). The task is to match the emotions at the bottom of the screen (Fig 17).

After finding the pairs, the pictures of emotion are again presented and the picture with a given emotion hasto be memorized. The patient then has to find the memorized emotion in the first set of pictures (Fig 17).

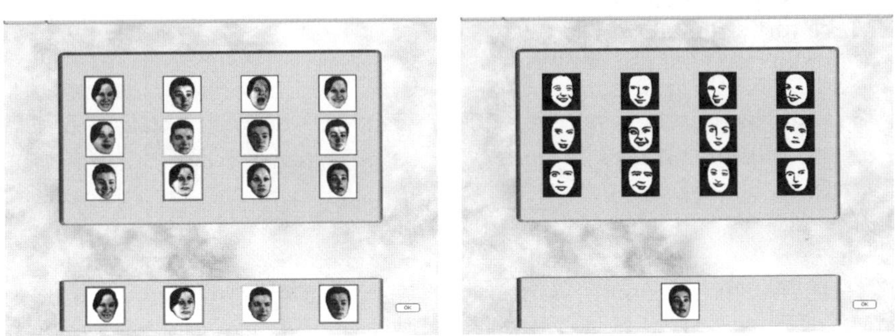

Fig. 17. Recognition of emotions

3.8.2 The framework and the database

The framework is responsible for requesting and changing the data of patients and neuropsychologists, creating a series of tasks it saves the steps of tasks into the database.

After logging in the neuropsychologist can:

- Browse among the results of a patient's former examinations
- Create a new series of tasks for the patient

In the diagnostic phase the neuropsychologist can change the task sequence any time he chooses another task to be the next.

In the database in addition to storing the personal data of the neuropsychologists and the patients, we store every step of the solution of every task and the comments of the neuropsychologist, so every solution can be reproduced and the patient's rehabilitation process followed.

The system is built to store the data of 100 -110 patients in a year assuming 20 – 25 examinations.

3.9. Results of the HELEN multimedia software

The program was tested with 6 healthy and 15 brain damaged patients.

During the examinations we received more information than in written tests, because we could save the steps taken by the patient. Therefore we could replay the steps and we give feedback to the patient.

The patient's idiosyncrasies are recorded, thus allowing his or her self-perceptions to change noticeably..

The results of healthy and sick patients differ a lot:

Sick people

- Need more time to observe
- Have a longer reaction time
- Require more help
- Make more mistakes

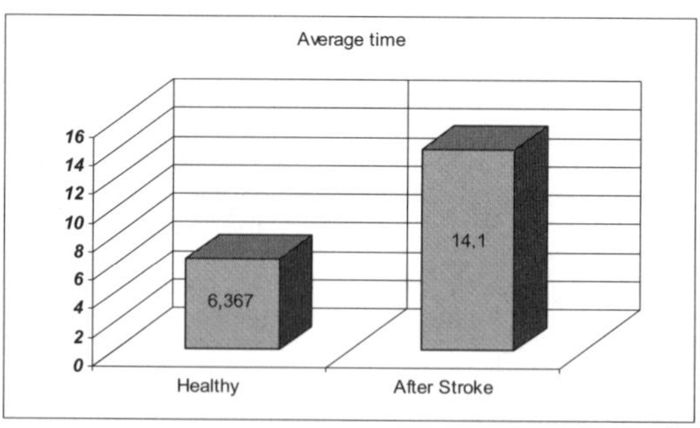

Fig. 18. Average time in seconds for Recognition tasks

Figure 18 shows a comparison of the average times taken by healthy people and patients after a stroke to solve the tasks of recognizing faces and recognizing emotions. Stroke Patients took twice as long as healthy people to solve tasks.

The damage of cognitive functions causes an increase in the number of steps in the tasks "How many pictures do you see?" and "Puzzle" (Fig. 19).

During the tests we realized that the experience of using computers plays an important role, so we needed to give the patients' time to practise.

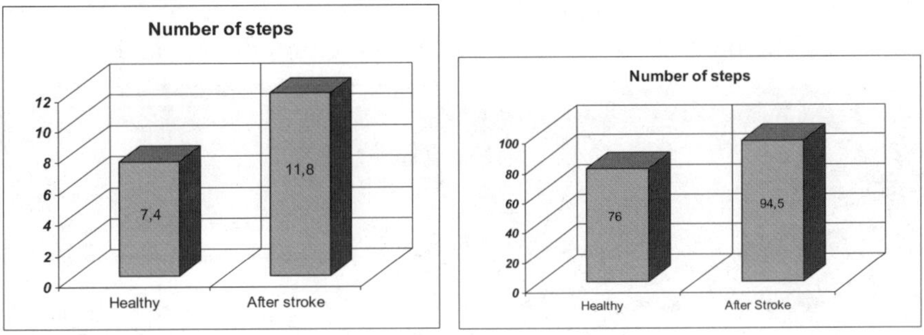

Fig. 19. (a): Number of steps of "How many pictures do you see?" (b): Number of steps of "Puzzle".

3.10 Program for aphasic patients

For aphasic patients we developed the "Word-instructor" software that teaches the aphasic patients the most important everyday words [70].

The programming was started after searching for simple figures and illustrations that were easy to identify. To begin with we had to consider that there were a lot of similar exercises. The program had to be finite. The number of the pictures visible on the screen is not the same in every task therefore we had to be careful of the size of each. The order in which they appeared was also important. The pictures are randomly arranged in every skill level of the program. In this way monotony is avoided. By using the interactivity of our software the computer gives the user information about correct or incorrect solutions. Both cases are marked with adequate figures and sound.

3.10.1 The introduction of the software

The program starts with a task being chosen. The user may not be able to use the software alone in this phase of the rehabilitation, so a teacher or a therapist's guidance is required. Answering the questions does not happen in a fixed order, so it is possible to begin the practice from his (or her) own skill level.

We took care to ensure interactive participation of the patient by ensuring each task required some manipulation. The number of the right answers isn't displayed with points but only with illustrating animations. The program is user friendly, it does not require special knowledge and everybody is able to understand how to use it in a few seconds.

3.10.2 The structure of the menu

There are three pictures in the main menu of the program (Fig. 20).

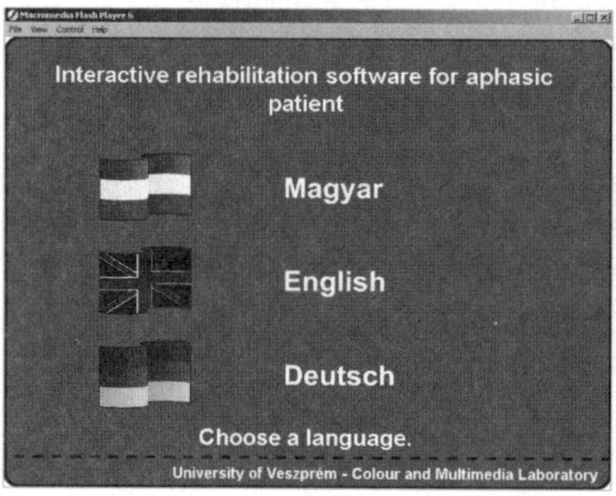

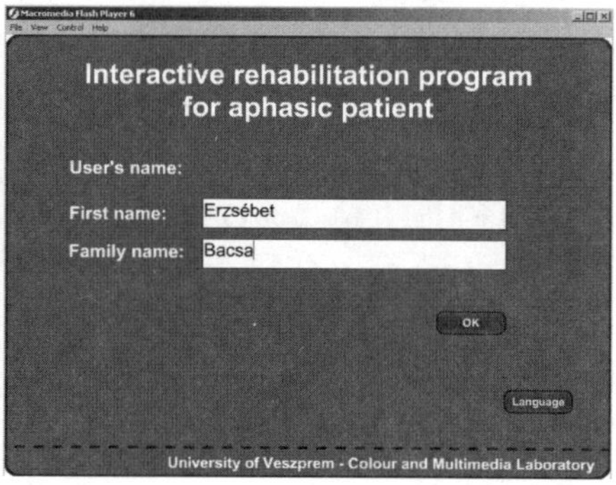

Fig. 20. Main menu

Fig. 21. Submenu - User's name

Here the patient or the teacher can choose from the language with a mouse click. The next step after choosing the language to give the user's first and family name. The user's name is required for further development of the records.

You can get into the next level only after filling in the User's name field. Then you can choose a room. (Fig. 22) The main task of the software is to teach the everyday words of the house or of the environment around to the house. In every submenu there are 4 skill levels (Fig. 23).

The first level acquaints the user with the objects of the room (Fig. 24). If the user points with the mouse to an object, the name of the object appears on the screen and it can be read. This first skill level trains the user's memory power.

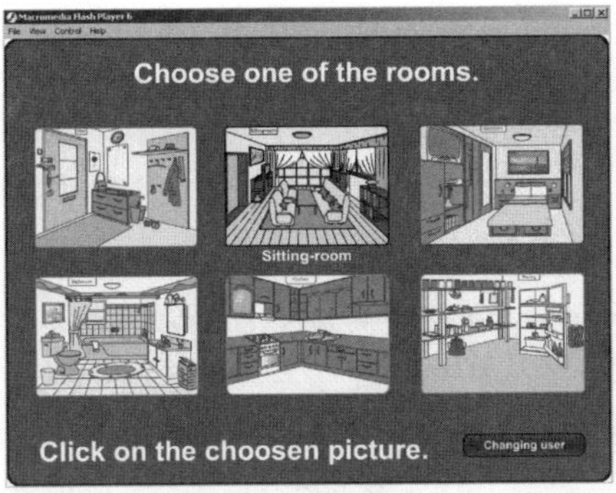

Fig. 22. Submenu – rooms

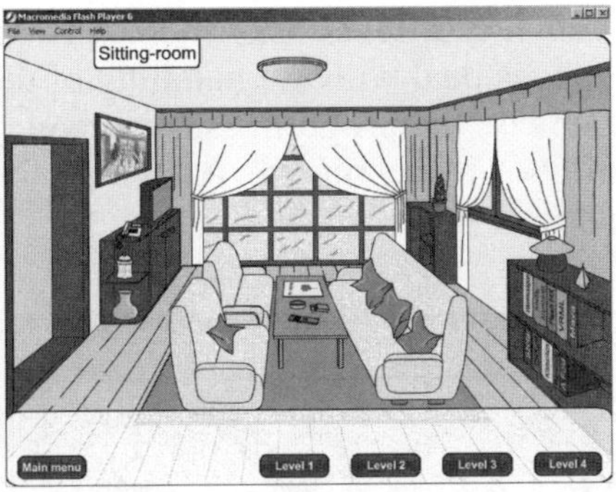

Fig. 23. Menu of the room

The second level shows an uncoloured picture. The program asks the user to show the name of objects (Fig. 25). If the user manages to find the object requested it becomes coloured. In this way the user can make the whole picture colourful. If the user is unsuccessful, the program sends an error message and the user can continue.

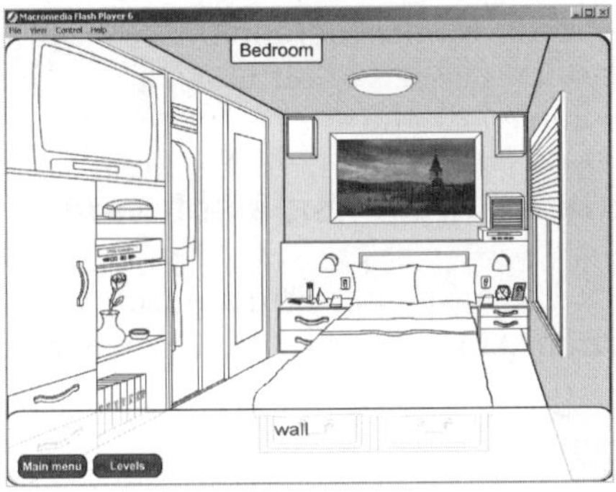

Fig. 24. 1st skill level

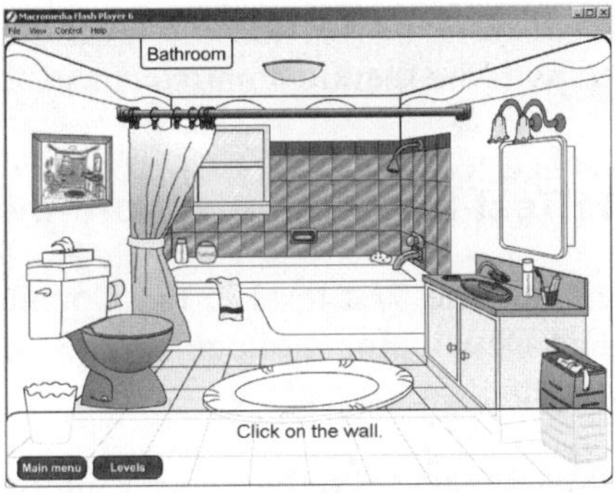

Fig. 25. 2nd skill level

The user's ability is also measured on the third level. The room used in the earlier task is in the background, but it is pale. (Fig. 26) The program shows three figures randomly and the user has to choose one by answering a question. This is essential to test if the patient is now able to identify the item used for the asked function. The real knowledge is examined at this level.

If the user could not answer, the program sends an error picture. This third level asks questions until the user or the teacher chooses another skill level.

The fourth level asks more difficult questions than the third level. The questions deal with the handling of the objects (Fig. 27). If the user can find the object, the program asks its name and the user has to write it into an input row on the screen. After the correct answer the program asks a new question.

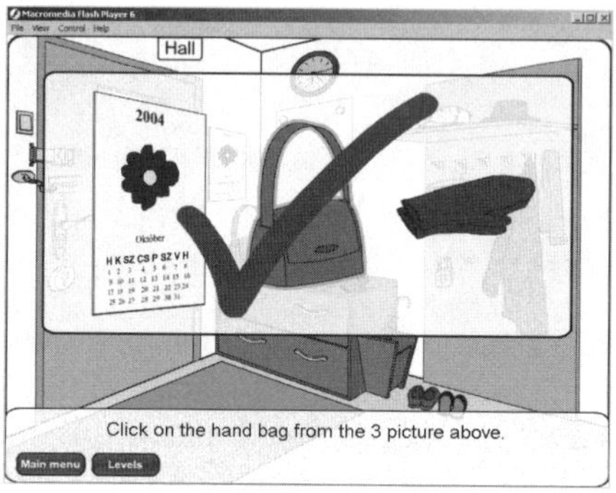
Hall
2004
Click on the hand bag from the 3 picture above.
Main menu
Levels

Fig. 26. 3rd skill level

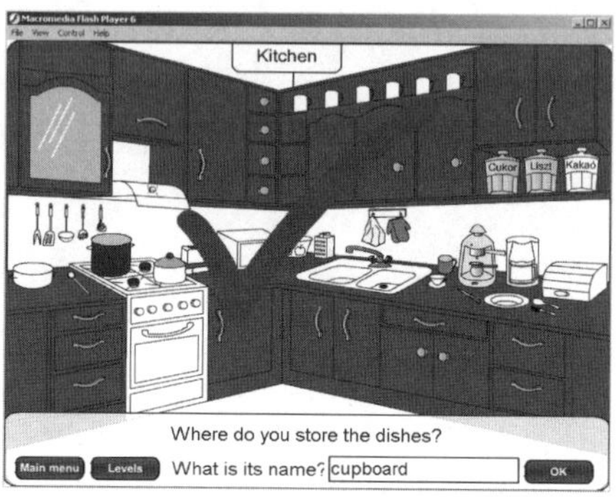

Fig. 27. 4th skill level

The starting level and the tasks are chosen by the therapist. They can be used with the therapist's assistance.

3.11 Test results of the Word-instructor multimedia software

We made the first tests in the Kozmutza Flora Special Primary School and Talent Developing College, where children with aphasia and other learning difficulties are educated.

We have tested only the user interface design so far.

One result of the first test is that the software is a useful device not only in the education of aphasic children but also children with severe learning difficulties. Moreover, it can be used easily by both the children and the teachers. Taking account of the advice of the teachers assisting us during the program development children need some motivating animation to reassure them of the correct answer and increase their interest in the subsequent items.

In the second step efficiency examinations were conducted not only in a school but in the National Centre of Brain Vein Diseases in Budapest too.

The psychologist's initial feedback was:

- The software needs a database.

- In the Hungarian language one distinguishes between addressing somebody by first name or family name. Grown ups are addressed normally by their family name.
- Adults do not require motivating exercises or tasks.

Five people with difficulties in naming objects have been tested up to now.

They managed to progress through levels 1-3 easily.

The 2nd task was the "painting" task. Column 1 of Table 5 shows the number of the objects that were found by the patients immediately. Column number 2 shows the number of the objects that were found by the patients at second trial, and so on. 91% of the objects were found at the first session. It was an easy task for every patient (Table 4).

Table 4: Number of correct answers at the 2nd level

Number of attempts	1	2	3	4	5	6	7	8	
1st person	29	4		1					
2nd person	30	2							
3rd person	8	1			1				
4th person	29								
5th person	28	2		1	1				
	124	9		2	2				137
%	91	7		1.5	1.5				

Why was every object not found immediately? Why were there 9% errors? Because these objects were very small or they were very hard to find. For example in the room: frame, candle, flower, cigarette, or in the bathroom: toothbrush, soap, soap-dish, body lotion. We are of the opinion that there were no mistakes.

Table 5: Number of correct answers at the 3rd level

Number of attempts	1	2	3	4	5	6	7	8	
1st person	14	1							
2nd person	25								
3rd person	12	1							
4th person	28								
5th person	28	2		1	1				
	107	4		1	1				113
%	94	4		1	1				

In the 3rd level the user was shown 3 objects. The task was to point to the requested object. Column 1 of Table 6 shows the number of objects that were found by the patients immediately. Column 2 shows the number of objects that were found by the patients at second trial, and so on. 94% of the objects were found at the first attempt (Table 5). It was also an easy task for every patient.

Here the patients had problems with long or compound words. For example: coffee table (in Hungarian it is even longer: dohányzóasztal) or videotape (in Hungarian: videókazetta).

The 4th level's task was the hardest of all. Here the patient had to answer and type the name of the requested object's. We can see in Table 6, only 44% of the tasks were solved immediately. Most of the questions were solved only at a second, third or later attempt..

Table 6: Number of the errors at the 4th level

Number of attempts	1	2	3	4	5	6	7	8	
1st person	1				1	1		1	
2nd person	6	2	1		1				
3rd person		1	1	2					
4th person	10	2	1	1		1	1		
5th person		1	2	1	1				
	17	6	5	4	3	2	1	1	39
%	44	15	13	10	8	5	2.5	2.5	

The problem here was not just the long or compound words, but also finding characters, mainly the accented letters. For example: gas-cooker = gáztűzhely, night-light = éjjelilámpa, oven – gloves = edényfogó kesztyű.

We want in the future to give some help in this task. For example going back to the 1st level, where the user can see the picture, and can point to the object. In this case he or she can read the name of the object. Perhaps it would be a very useful help if synonyms could also be accepted by the software. It is our future plan.

4. Future

The recent revolution in telemedicine, i.e. telecommunication, multimedia, and information technologies, to provide and support health care when distance separates participants and doctors, offers an opportunity to address the problem of the unequal geographical distribution of physicians and the lack of health care services in rural and urban districts. Many predict that telemedicine will have a significant impact on the delivery of care in the future; some predict that telemedicine will revolutionize how care is delivered. As these technologies become more developed and widely disseminated, physicians will probably be able to manage larger numbers of patients. Patient management will be facilitated by new information support systems designed for use by both physicians and patients. For these reasons it has been predicted that this increase in productivity will result in the need for fewer physicians, both generalists and sub-specialists, to meet health care demands [71].

Competition in the health care industry has encouraged the dissemination of telemedicine. Integrated delivery systems are aggressively seeking competitive advantages and have been willing to explore the use of new technologies to support this goal. Ongoing advances in telemedicine (i.e. telecommunication, multimedia, and information technologies) are likely to change dramatically how paediatric care is delivered in the future. In addition to enhancing paediatricians' efforts to monitor and improve quality of care, telemedicine offers the potential to increase efficiency and to enhance communication between paediatricians and other members of the child health care team. It is also likely that these technologies will play a role in reshaping the relationships among physicians, their patients, and other members of the multidisciplinary care team [72].

Current speech recognition systems have evolved technologically to begin having an impact in human computer interface (HCI) designs that can be used by persons with motor disabilities. A real-time user friendly programming HCI is able to convert voice commands into computer actions [73]. These voice controlled HCI systems would be the optimal support solutions for people with motor disability.

5. Conclusion

In the last two decades multimedia has become an important tool in preventive and assistive healthcare. The physicians' nurses and patients use such applications too. For healthcare staff multimedia applications are used for saving and sending images, helping to make diagnoses, education, further training and teleconferencing. Multimedia is an information tool, education and rehabilitation tool also for patients.

Multimedia can be an important tool to teach children. The teaching of disabled children with multimedia tools is an important area of application. We have selected the area of producing multimedia games for partially sighted-, hearing impaired and motor impaired children because here the multimedia games can be used very effectively. It is an important area of application. These games can be used both in individual and small-group teaching. They can also be given to parents to use with their children.

The computer can be used, with the help of appropriate software, in the therapy of amblyopia and in the therapy of hearing impaired patients. We are convinced that such games can help the development visus of children's vision and learning new words. We have first considered the needs and, after getting first reactions from the teachers, have developed the programs in such a form that they can be used effectively.

The teachers gave a summarised opinion about our software for hearing impaired children. The general experiences of the teachers are the following:

- Children can use both software programs by themselves very easily and they enjoy using them, which is a very important factor from the point of view of efficiency.
- The system is a useful tool for teachers in individual linguistic training. It provides possibility of training in small groups too as well as the pupils using the system themselves and practising alone.
- The simple child-like drawings are preferred to professional figures.
- Most hearing impaired children also require sounds.

To sum up, the children used the software with pleasure and success; they wished that more school teaching material was like these software programmes.

Helen for stroke patients and the world-instructor for aphasic patients
The group of interactive computer controlled rehabilitation programs makes it possible to reveal the individual changes in the mental capacity of the patient, and by doing this get new information on the cognitive functioning of the patient or group of patients.

The information in the database reveals further data on the individual path followed by the patient, this can provide information on his/her typical behaviour and how he or she recognizes something, thus giving us further insight in the sequencing of perceptions.

The interactive software package was designed so that at the diagnostic phase the patient uses it in the presence of the neuropsychologist. Using the other tasks he/she can learn and improve his/her abilities by themselves.

The Helen software enables the examination and rehabilitation of stroke patients in such a way, that it encourages the patient to look for a way out in situations that could lead to failure. He/she can choose one of the existing possibilities, but he/she always controls the process. It is important that using a computer should not become mechanical, the patient should not depend on the computer, but the scale of his/her problem solving strategies should become wider. With its help under the lead of a neuropsychologist the patients can find their own pathway during rehabilitation, which can be important to their personal self-esteem. On the other hand we can get the answers to the question: 'what are the most important criteria from the viewpoint of the possibility of cognitive rehabilitation?'

The other program we have discussed in this paper can help further in the rehabilitation or it can also be used as a stand-alone rehabilitation tool.

In this chapter we have discussed the role of multimedia in healthcare. We saw that multimedia systems are becoming increasingly important in preventive and assistive healthcare. There will be more and more 3D applications and animations in the forthcoming multimedia software. These become very similar to virtual reality applications, a topic to be discussed in the next chapter.

References

1. http://www.scala.com/multimedia/multimedia-definition.html
2. Collen M.F., A Vision of Health Care and Informatics in 2008, Journal of the American Medical Informatics Association 1999;6(1):1-5.
3. Klar R., Selected Impressions on the Beginning of the Electronic Medical Record and Patient Information, Methods of Information in Medicine 2004; 43: 537-542.
4. Balch D.C., Tichenor J.M., Telemedicine Expanding the Scope of Health Care Information, Journal of the American Medical Informatics Association 1997; 4(1):1-5.
5. Goede P.A., Lauman J.R., Cochel C., Katzman G.L., Morton D.A., Albertine K.H., A Methodology and Implementation for Annotating Digital Images for Context-appropriate Use in an Academic Health Care Environment, Journal of the American Medical Informatics Association 2004; 11(1): 29 - 41.
6. Brinkley J.F., Rosse C., The Digital Anatomist Distributed Framework and Its Applications to Knowledge-based Medical Imaging, Journal of the American Medical Informatics Association 1997;4(3):165-183.
7. Lowe H.J., Antipov I., Hersh W., Smith C.A., Mailhot M., Automated Semantic Indexing of Imaging Reports to Support Retrieval of Medical Images in the Multimedia Electronic Medical Record, Methods of Information in Medicine 1999; 38: 303-307.
8. Bui A.A.T., McNitt-Gray M.F., Goldin J.G., Cardenas A.F., Aberle D.R., Problem-oriented Prefetching for an Integrated Clinical Imaging Workstation, Journal of the American Medical Informatics Association 2001;8(3): 242-253.
9. Wong S.T.C., Soo Hoo K. Jr, Knowlton R.C., Laxer K.D., Cao X., Hawkins R.A., Dillon W.P., Arenson R.L., Design and Applications of a Multimodality

Image Data Warehouse Framework, Journal of the American Medical Informatics Association 2002;9(3):239-254.
10. McCullagh P. J., McAllister H. G., Howard R., Hong Neo L., Paradigms for Recording Cognitive Brain Electrical Activity, Methods of Information in Medicine 2001;40:184-189.
11. Jordan D.A., McKeown K.R., Concepcion K.J., Feiner S.K., Hatzivassiloglou V., Generation and Evaluation of Intraoperative Inferences for Automated Health Care Briefings on Patient Status After Bypass Surgery, Journal of the American Medical Informatics Association 2001;8(3):267-280.
12. Chun J., Kim H, Lee S., Choi J., Cho H., A DBMS-based Medical Teleconferencing System, Journal of the American Medical Informatics Association 2001;8(5):460-467.
13. Nenov V., Klopp J., Remote analysis of physiological data from neurosurgical ICU patients, Journal of the American Medical Informatics Association 1996;3(5):318-327.
14. Ketchell D.S., Freedman M.M., Jordan W.E., Lightfoot E.M., Heyano S, Libbey P.A., Willow: a uniform search interface, Journal of the American Medical Informatics Association 1996;3(1):27-37.
15. Humphreys B.L., Electronic Health Record Meets Digital Library: A New Environment for Achieving an Old Goal, Journal of the American Medical Informatics Association 2000;7(5):444-452.
16. Shifman M.A., Sayward F.G., Mattie M.E., Miller P.L., Exploring Issues of Quality of Service in a Next Generation Internet Testbed: A Case Study Using PathMaster, Journal of the American Medical Informatics Association 2002;9(5):491-499.
17. Jakobovits R.M., Rosse C., Brinkley J.F., WIRM An Open Source Toolkit for Building Biomedical Web Applications, Journal of the American Medical Informatics Association 2002; 9(6):557-570.
18. Chan T.C., Killeen J., Griswold W., Lenert L., Information Technology and Emergency Medical Care during Disasters, Academic Emergency Medicine 2004; 11(11): 1229 - 1236.
19. Maglaveras N., Chouvarda I., Koutkias V., Meletiadis S., Haris K., Balas E.A., Information Technology Can Enhance Quality in Regional Health Delivery, Methods of Information in Medicine 2002; 41: 393-400.
20. Kinzie M.B., Cohn W.F., Julian M.F., Knaus W.A., A User-centered Model for Web Site Design: Needs Assessment, User Interface Design, and Rapid Prototyping, Journal of the American Medical Informatics Association 2002;9(4):320-330.
21. Williams R.G., Stein L.D., Leslie L.K., Training Pediatricians for the Evolving Generalist-Specialist Interface in the Managed Care Era, Pediatrics Vol. 101 No. 4 Supplement April 1998, pp. 779-784.
22. Athreya B.H., Cheh M.L., Kingsland L.C.III, Computer-assisted Diagnosis of Pediatric Rheumatic Diseases, Pediatrics, 1998, Vol. 102 No. 4 pp. 48.
23. Okada Y., Haruki Y., Ogushi Y., Disaster Drills and Continuous Medical Education using Satellite-based Internet, Methods of Information in Medicine 2000; 39: 343-347.

24. Fanaroff A.F., Challenges for neonatology and neonatologists. J Perinatol 1999; 19:329.
25. Halamek L.P., Kaegi D.M., Gaba D.M., Sowb Y.A., Bradford C. Smith, Brian E. Smith, and Steven K. Howard, Time for a New Paradigm in Pediatric Medical Education: Teaching Neonatal Resuscitation in a Simulated Delivery Room Environment, Pediatrics, 2000, Vol. 106 No. 4, pp 45.
26. Hillenbrand K.M., Larsen P.G., Effect of an Educational Intervention About Breastfeeding on the Knowledge, Confidence, and Behaviors of Pediatric Resident Physicians, Pediatrics, 2002, Vol. 110 No. 5, pp.59.
27. Friedl R., Klas W., WestermannU., Rose T., Tremper J., Stracke S., Gödje O., Hannekum A., Preisack M.B., The CardioOP-Data Clas (CDC) Development and Application of a Thesaurus for Content Management and Multi-User Teleteaching in Cardiac Surgery, Methods of Information in Medicine 2003; 42: 68-78.
28. Dev P., Montgomery K., Senger S., Heinrichs W.L., Srivastava S., Waldron K., Simulated Medical Learning Environments on the Internet, Journal of the American Medical Informatics Association 2002;9(5):437-447.
29. Temkin B., Acosta E., Hatfield P., Onal E., Tong A., Web-based Three-dimensional Virtual Body Structures: W3D-VBS, Journal of the American Medical Informatics Association 2002;9(5):425-436.
30. Tirado-Ramos A., Hu J., Lee K.P., Information Object Definition–based Unified Modeling Language Representation of DICOM Structured Reporting: A Case Study of Transcoding DICOM to XML, Journal of the American Medical Informatics Association 2002;9(1):63-72.
31. Dolin R.H., Alschuler L., Beebe C., Biron P.V., Boyer S.L., Essin D., Kimber E., Lincoln T., Mattison J.E., The HL7 Clinical Document Architecture, Journal of the American Medical Informatics Association 2001;8(6):552-569.
32. Lenert L.A., Soetikno R.M., Automated Computer Interviews to Elicit Utilities: Potential Applications in the Treatment of Deep Venous Thrombosis, Journal of the American Medical Informatics Association 1997;4(1):49-56.
33. Tetzlaff L., Consumer Informatics in Chronic Illness, Journal of the American Medical Informatics Association 1997; 4(4):285-300.
34. McRoy S.W., Liu-Perez A., Ali S.S., Interactive Computerized Health Care Education, Journal of the American Medical Informatics Association 1998;5(4):347-356.
35. Homer C., Susskind O., Alpert H.R., Owusu C., Schneider L., Rappaport L.A., Rubin D.H., An Evaluation of an Innovative Multimedia Educational Software Program for Asthma Management: Report of a Randomized, Controlled Trial, Pediatrics, 2000, Vol. 106 No. 1, pp. 210-215., available at:http://pediatrics.aappublications.org/cgi/content/full/106/1/S1/210
36. Krishna S., Francisco B.D., Balas E.A., König P., Graff G.R., Madsen R.W., Internet-Enabled Interactive Multimedia Asthma Education Program: A Randomized Trial, Pediatrics, 2003, Vol. 111 No. pp. 503-510.
37. Shegog R., Bartholomew L.K., Parcel G.S., Sockrider M.M., Mâsse L., Abramson S.L., Impact of a Computer-assisted Education Program on Factors Related to Asthma Self-management Behavior, Journal of the American Medical Informatics Association 2001;8(1):49-61.

38. Chambers M.G., Connor S.L., McGonigle M., Diver M.G., Multimedia Software to Help Caregivers Cope, Journal of the American Medical Informatics Association 2003;10(5):504-511.
39. Feeney Mahoney D., Tarlow B.J., Jones R.N., Sandaire J., Effects of a Multimedia Project on Users' Knowledge about Normal Forgetting and Serious Memory Loss, Journal of the American Medical Informatics Association 2002;9(4):383-394.
40. Gray J.E., Safran C., Davis R.B., Pompilio-Weitzner G., Stewart J.E., Zaccagnini L., Pursley D., Baby CareLink: Using the Internet and Telemedicine to Improve Care for High-Risk Infants, Pediatrics, 2000, Vol. 106 No. 6, pp. 1318-1324.
41. Muñoz-Furlong A., Daily Coping Strategies for Patients and Their Families, Pediatrics, 2003, Vol. 111 No. 6, pp. 1654-1661.
42. Porter S.C., Kohane I.S., Goldmann D.A., Parents as Partners in Obtaining the Medication History, Journal of the American Medical Informatics Association 2005;12(3):299-305.
43. Brodin, J. Opportunities and obstacles. Computer play for vhildren with profound intellectual impairment and multiple disabilities. Assistive Technologies – Added Value to the Quality of Life, Marinek et al. (Eds.) IOS Press, 2001, pp. 349-352.
44. Blenkhorn P.L., Microcomputer Software Using a Touch Sensitive Screen, The British Journal of Special Education. December, 4, 161.
45. Blenkhorn P.L., Tobin M.J., Report on computer hardware in schools and units for the visually handicapped, University of Bimingham, Research Centre fort he Education of the Visually Handicapped.
46. Spencer S., Ross M., Tobin M.J., Blenkhorn P.L., Centre Computer Base for Visually handicapped children, students and adults, The British Journal of Visual Impairment, V, pp. 67-69.
47. Blenkhorn P.L., Evans G., Using a multimedai computer to support visual asesment and training of early visual skills for children with profound and multiple disabilities, Assistive Technologies – Added Value to the Quality of Life, Marinek et al. (Eds.) IOS Press, 2001, pp. 364-368.
48. Brodin J., Jonson U., Computer play centres for children with disabilities, International Journal of Rehabilitation Research, 23, pp. 125-128.
49. Batusic M., Burger F., Miesenberger K., Stöger B., Special problems of blind people in accessing mathematical information. Accessed from http://www.aib.uni-linz.ac.at/PAPER1/PAPER.HTML
50. Archambault D. and al. TIM, Tactile Interactive Multimedia computer games for visually impaired children, May 2000. This project is founded by the European Comission – Information Society Technologies, ref. IST-2000-25298.
51. Archambault D., Burger D., Sable S., The TIM Project: Tactile Interactive Multimedai computer games for blind and visually impaired children, Assistive Technologies – Added Value to the Quality of Life, Marinek et al. (Eds.) IOS Press, 2001, pp. 359-363.
52. Sablé S., Archambault D., Blindstation: a Game Platform Adapted to Visually Impaired Children, Assistive Technologies – Shaping the Future, Craddock et al. (Eds.) IOS Press, 2003, pp. 232 -236.

53. Ruseckaite R., Lukauskiene R., Assistive technologies for children. Restoration of visual perception functions, Assistive Technologies – Added Value to the Quality of Life, Marinek et al. (Eds.) IOS Press, 2001, pp. 369-373.
54. Velleman E., van Tol R., Huiberts S., Verwey H., 3D Shooting Games, Multimodal Games, Sound Games and More Working Examples of the Future of Games for the Blind, Computers Helping People with Special Needs, Zagler at al. (Eds.) Springer Press, 2002, pp. 257-263.
55. Beck C., Interface für Kommunikationssysteme für Schwerstbehinderte basierend auf IR Sensoren. Diplomarbeit, TU Wien.
56. Kobayashi M., Watanabe T., A tactile display system equipped with a pointing device – MIMIZU. Computers Helping People with Special Needs, Miesenberger at al. (Eds.) Springer Press, 2002, pp.527-534.
57. Minagawa H., Kobayashi M., Nishioka T., Miyoshi S., A Character Based Communication System as a Universal Design, Especially for the Visual and the Hearing Impaired, Proc. Computers Helping People with Special Needs, Vollmar and Wagner (Eds.), pp. 489-495., Kalsruhe, Deutschland, 17-21. July. 2000.
58. Kobayashi M., Minagawa H., Nishioka T., Miyoshi S., Chating System that Supports Communication between the Visually and the Hearing Impaired, Proc. Computers Helping People with Special Needs, Vollmar and Wagner (Eds.), pp. 497-502., Kalsruhe, Deutschland, 17-21. July. 2000.
59. Coursant-Moreau A., Crépy H., Destombes F., LIPCOM: An IBM Research Project to Help Speech Perception by Deaf Persons, Proc. Computers Helping People with Special Needs, Vollmar and Wagner (Eds.), pp. 127-134., Kalsruhe, Deutschland, 17-21. July. 2000.
60. Alcantud F., Asensi M.C., Ferer A.M., Romero R., Multimedia based instruction of reading comprehension for deaf people: Experiment results, Proc. Computers Helping People with Special Needs, Vollmar Wagner (Eds.), pp. 579-586. Kalsruhe, Deutschland, 17-21. July 2000.
61. Pimlott C., Blenkhorn P., Evans D.G., An Alternative Interface Paradigm for GUIs, Proc. Computers Helping People with Special Needs, Vollmar and Wagner (Eds.), pp. 67-73., Kalsruhe, Deutschland, 17-21. July. 2000.
62. Ferrer A., Romero R., Alcantud F., Analysis of disabled user regquirements for a web browsing scanning selection system, Proc. Computers Helping People with Special Needs, Vollmar and Wagner (Eds.), pp. 571-578., Kalsruhe, Deutschland, 17-21. July 2000.
63. Ferrer A., Romero R., Alcantud F., Web accessibility for people with motor impairments. Case studies, Proc. Computers Helping People with Special Needs, Vollmar and Wagner (Eds.), pp. 595-602., Kalsruhe, Deutschland, 17-21. July 2000.
64. Panek P., Beck C., Mina S., Seisenbacher G., Zagler W.L., Technical Assistence for Motor- and Multiple Disabled Children – Some Long Term Experiences, Computers Helping People with Special Needs, Miesenberger at al. (Eds.) Springer Press, 2002, pp. 181-188.
65. Spaniol M., Springer L., Klamma R., Jarke M., SOCRATES: Barrier Free Communities of Aphasics on the Internet, Computers Helping People with Special Needs, Miesenberger at al. (Eds.) Springer Press, 2004, pp. 1024-1031.

66. Sik Lányi C., Lányi Zs: Multimedia Program for Training of Vision of Children, Journal of Information Technology Education, Volume 2, pp. 279-290.
67. Sik Lányi C., Váry Á., Sik A. ,Nemetz A., Geiszt Z, Multimedia Programs for Children with Hearing Difficulties, Computers Helping People with Special Needs, Miesenberger at al. (Eds.) Springer Press, 2004, pp. 14-21.
68. Sik Lányi C., Molnár Lányi Á.: Psychological and pedagogic testing of handicapped children with locomotion disorder using multimedia programs, Proc. 3rd International Conference on Disability, Virtual Reality and Associated Technologies, in Sharkey, Ceserani, Pugnetti and Rizzo (Eds), pp. 99-106., Algero, Sardinia, 23-25. Sept. 2000.
69. Sik Lányi C., Szabó J., Páll A., Pataky I., Computer-Controlled Cognitive Diagnostics and Rehabilitation Method for Stroke Patients, ERCIM News No. 61, April 2005 pp. 53-54.
70. Sik Lányi C., Bacsa E., Mátrai R., Kosztyán Zs., Pataky I., The Design Question of Development of Multimedia Educational Software for Aphasia Patients, Computers Helping People with Special Needs, Miesenberger at al. (Eds.) Springer Press, 2004, pp. 6-13.
71. DeAngelis C., Feigin R., DeWitt T., First L.R., Jewett E.A., Kelch R., Chesney R.W., Mulvey H.J., Simon J.L., Alden E.R., Final Report of the FOPE II Pediatric Workforce Workgroup, Pediatrics, 2000, Vol. 106 No. 5, pp. 1245-1255.
72. The Future of Pediatric Education II: Organizing Pediatric Education to Meet the Needs of Infants, Children, Adolescents, and Young Adults in the 21st Century, Pediatrics, 2000, Vol. 105 No. 1, pp. 163-21
73. Adjouadi M., Landestoy D., Ayala M., Tischer W., A Real-Time Voice Controlled Human Computer Interface to Help Persons with Motor Disability, Computers Helping People with Special Needs, Miesenberger at al. (Eds.) Springer Press, 2004, pp. 804-812.

3 Virtual Reality in Healthcare

Cecília Sik Lányi
Faculty of Information Technology
University of Veszprém
H-8200 Veszprém, Egyetem u. 10., Hungary

Abstract. In our modern 21st century, daily life would be unthinkable without computers. Multimedia and virtual reality are useful for people with special needs. This chapter presents a general overview of the use of virtual reality in medical informatics, rehabilitation and assistive & preventive healthcare.

1. Introduction

Virtual reality is being applied to a wide range of medical areas, including medical education/training, surgery and diagnostic assistance for heath staff. For patients it is used for their rehabilitation and training.

1.1. Definition of VE and VR

Virtual Environment (VE): A synthetic, spatial (usually 3D) world seen from a first-person's point of view. The view in a VE is under the real-time control of the user.

Virtual Reality (VR) is synonymous with VE. We use the term VE in this article because the term VR is associated with unrealistic hype generated by the media [1].

Multi-sensory VEs are closed-loop systems comprised of humans, computers, and the interfaces through which continuous streams of information flow. More specifically, VEs are distinguished from other simulator systems by their capacity to portray three-dimensional (3D) spatial information in a variety of modalities, their ability to exploit users' natural input behaviours for human-computer interaction, and their potential to "immerse" the user in the virtual world [2].

VR is a part of computer science, that allows computer based models of the real world to be generated, and provides humans with a means to interact with these models through new human-computer interfaces. It can either be immersive, where the user feels physically present in the VE, typically

C.S. Lányi: *Virtual Reality in Healthcare*, Studies in Computational Intelligence (SCI) **19**, 87–116 (2006)
www.springerlink.com

using a head-mounted display or non immersive, where a handheld interface allows interaction with objects on a computer screen.

2. VR for the healthcare staff

How can we categorize VR in healthcare? These applications are used by physicians' nurses and patients too. For healthcare staff VR applications are used to help make diagnoses, for education, further training and teleconferencing. VR is an information and, education tool and rehabilitation tool for patients. The main question is how we can develop such VR applications. How can the user needs, the contents and the technical possibilities be harmonised?

2.1. For the healthcare staff training and education

In the medical education field, VR opens up new realms in the teaching of medicine and creates new effective learning procedures for students. In contrast with the expensive immersive virtual reality learning environment (VRLE) such as Cave Automatic Virtual Environment (CAVE), ImmersaDesk, Virtual Reality Modelling Language (VRML) technology provides an inexpensive and simple way to create such an environment and can easily be deployed in the classroom.

Modern medicine is evolving rapidly with new and better medical techniques being elaborated. But the new procedures tend to become more and more complex. There is no better way for medical students to learn than to practise. But training with live patients is very risky. So this is why virtual reality (VR) technique is being widely applied.

Many innovative tools have emerged from education research, but we are still struggling to determine how those tools can be best used in the pursuit of the educational mission [3]. Advances in mainstream education research, such as adaptive hypermedia [4], intelligent tutoring systems [5], simulations [6, 7], and decision support systems for education [8] need to be applied, evaluated, and validated in biomedical environments. We set out some of these innovative VR tools in detail:

Learning anatomy and surgical procedures requires both a conceptual understanding of three-dimensional anatomy and a hands-on manipulation of tools and tissue. Such virtual resources are not available widely, are expensive, and may be culturally unacceptable. Simulation technology, using high-performance computers and graphics, permits realistic real-time display of anatomy. Haptics technology supports the ability to probe and feel this virtual anatomy through the use of virtual tools. The Internet permits world-wide access to resources. At Stanford University the researchers have brought together high-performance servers and high-bandwidth communication using the Next Generation Internet and complex bimanual haptics to simulate a tool-based learning environment for wide use [7].

Dornan at al. [9] described qualitative analysis of students' requirements in their medical skills curriculum and proposed a web-based presentation of clinical skills curriculum. The Anatomic VisualizeR is a VR-based environment for the teaching and learning of clinical anatomy initially developed by the University of California [10].

Major efforts are being made to improve the teaching of human anatomy to foster cognition of visuospatial relationships. The Visible Human Project of the National Library of Medicine makes it possible to create virtual reality-based applications for teaching anatomy. Integration of traditional cadaver and illustration-based methods with Internet-based simulations brings us closer to achieve the goal of efficient education [11].

At the University of Michigan user data and information about anatomy education were used to guide development of a learning environment that is efficient and effective. The research question focused on how to design instructional software suitable for the educational goals of different groups of users of the Visible Human data set. Information about learning challenges and processes was gathered to define essential anatomy teaching strategies [12].

Jianfeng Lu and co-workers discussed a system that is used for education in medicine using inexpensive equipment. The system is implemented with ready-to-use techniques such as VRML and visualization toolkit (VTK). They developed their prototype of VRLE system at the Zhejiang University [13].

In April 2000 the National Library of Medicine [14] posted a beta test site titled "AnatLine" providing a variety of new resources derived from The National Library of Medicine's Visible Human Project. The implica-tions of three dimensionality for enhancing anatomical understanding from viewing computer models was pointed out [15, 16], and interactive 3D les-sons have been incorporated into the curriculum at UCSD and Uniformed Services University of the Health Sciences [17]. The AnatLine database provides users and developers with significant "value added" compared to the raw CCD images previously available. The color images derived from the 70mm film are spectacular in the detail which can be observed, and their availability is beneficial. However, availability of the segmentations of structures of interest from the cross sectional data is the most exciting, since this time consuming process is the main limitation in the creation of a collection of 3D Visible Human models. Downloading, analysing and expanding the Anat-

Line VHI files results in cross sectional masks, which are easily contoured and reconstructed into surface models with minimal effort using appropriate software. Segmentations have been specified at several granularities, so that one can quickly construct models of the entire heart, or of individual chambers, or of the vertebral column or of an individual vertebra. The database provides a search engine which enables the user to learn what structures are available, and in what collections of subparts or larger systems. The database is designed to accommodate expansion, and alternative segmentations will likely be added. The availability of rendered images (TIFF files) is useful, though 3D surfaces and/or their VRML representations provide a much greater potential for a wider variety of uses [14].

Virtual reality based surgical simulator systems offer a very elegant possibility of enriching and enhancing traditional education. A wide range of VR simulator systems have been proposed and implemented in the past few years. Some of them are restricted to purely diagnostic endoscopical investigations, while others, for example, allow the training of surgical procedures for laparoscopic, arthroscopic, or radiological interventions [18].

These applications were successfully applied in the real teaching and learning procedure. The field of VR in medical education is gaining recognition and various efforts have been undertaken to improve medical education and training using them. The VR-based education and training will be the principal platform in the new century.

2.2. For making diagnosis

The 1998 Scientific Symposium of the American College of Medical Informatics (ACMI) was devoted to developing visions for the future of health care and biomedicine as well as to establishing a strategic agenda for health and biomedical informatics in support of those visions. The fo-cus of this symposium was prompted by the many major changes currently underway in health care delivery, education, and research, as well as in our health and biomedical enterprises, and by the constantly increasing role of information technology in both shaping and enabling these changes. The three ambitious goals developed for 2008 are a virtual health care data-bank, a national health care knowledge base, and a personal clinical health record [19]. We are nearing the achievement of these goals, we already have a virtual health care databank and also a personal clinical health record. In our opinion , we (the patients) need in the future in our personal clinical health record not only the dry data and facts of monitoring our body, but also to see in 3D VR the problem and its possible solution.

In the Medical University of Lübeck a system has been created for the virtual planning of hip operations with endoprosthetic reconstruction and its application in bone tumour surgery. The system enables the simulation of the operation and the construction of a custom-made implant related to the chosen resection planes and the patient's anatomy. During the planning process integrated virtual reality techniques facilitate the interaction with the three-dimensional (3D) medical objects. Stereo viewing improves the perception of the 3D nature of bone structures and tumours. In comparison to conventional planning procedures, different operation strategies and their influence on the geometry of the custom-made endoprosthesis can be easily compared. Furthermore, the combination of multi-modal image information (CT and MR) enables an accurate 3D visualization of the bone tumour within the bone [20].

Mazziotta et al. described the development of a four-dimensional atlas and reference system that includes both macroscopic and microscopic information on structure and function of the human brain in persons between the ages of 18 and 90 years. Examples of applications of the approach were described for the normal brain in both adults and children as well as in patients with schizophrenia. This project should provide new insights into the relationship between microscopic and macroscopic structure and function in the human brain and should have important implications in basic neuroscience, clinical diagnostics, and cerebral disorders [21].

A medical teleconferencing system was designed in Korea that is integrated with a multimedia patient database and incorporates easy-to-use tools and functions to effectively support collaborative work between physicians in remote locations. The design provides a virtual workspace that allows physicians to collectively view various kinds of patient data. By integrating the teleconferencing function into this workspace, physicians are able to conduct conferences using the same interface and have real-time access to the database during conference sessions. The prototype uses a high-speed network test bed and a manually created substitute for the integrated patient database [22].

A grid-like computing environment was successfully implemented on a wide-area cluster system. The system can be applied to interactive simulation, where a cluster is used for high-performance computations, while a dedicated immersive interactive environment (CAVE) offers visualization and user interaction. Design considerations for the construction of dynamic exploration environments using such a system are discussed, in particular the use of intelligent agents for coordination. A case study of simulated abdominal vascular reconstruction is subsequently presented: the results of computed tomography or magnetic resonance imaging of a patient are displayed in CAVE, and a surgeon can evaluate the possible treatments by performing the surgeries virtually and analysing the resulting blood flow which is simulated [23].

Poliakov et al. described a client-server approach to three-dimensional (3-D) visualization of neuroimaging data, which enables researchers to visualize, manipulate, and analyze large brain imaging datasets over the Internet. All computationally intensive tasks are done by a graphics server that loads and processes image volumes and 3-D models, renders 3-D scenes, and sends the results back to the client [24].

A paediatrician must be able to manage clinical information using current information and technology to its full advantage. In addition, computerized systems for shared decision-making and the Internet will empower patients to take an active part in their care, enhancing their confidence. How these systems will impact on practices in the near future will depend on provider willingness to allow the traditional doctor-patient roles to become more reciprocal. These are behaviours that will need to be modelled for physicians-in-training [25].

A further typical use of VR is in surgical simulation and planning. There are a lot of publications in this field [26, 27, 28, 29]. A useful new tool is the virtual endoscopy. Virtual endoscopy is a new procedure that fuses computed tomography with advanced techniques for rendering three-dimensional images to produce views of the organ similar to chose obtained during real endoscopy [30, 31, 32].

A technique that can lead us into the future is perhaps the following: There has been speculation about virtual endoscopic capabilities since the early 1970's, as dramatized in the science fiction movie "Fantastic Voyage", the recent availability of the Visible Human Datasets (VHD) from the National Library of Medicine, coupled with the development of computer algorithms to accurately and rapidly render high resolution images in 3-D and perform fly-through instead of inserting long instruments (endoscopes of any kind) into a patient, has provided modern realization of these capabilities. The VHD provides a rich opportunity to help advance this important new methodology from theory to practice [33].

In the future we can expect the development of different VR dynamic models illustrating how various organs and systems move during normal or diseased states, or how they respond to various externally applied forces. In all these cases VR simulators allow the acquisition of necessary technical skills required for the proper operational procedure [34].

3. For the patients

VR is an information, education and rehabilitation tool of the patients. VR is starting to play an important role in clinical practice and in clinical psychology, but it could be as a support tool in preventive healthcare too.

3.1. VR as an information and education tool for the patients

Internet based consultations between specialists at centres of excellence and referring doctors can contribute to patient care through recommendations for new treatment and timely access to specialist knowledge. Kedar and co-workers described such a consultation system. Although change in diagnosis occurred in only a few cases, the prognostic and therapeutic implications for these patients might have been be profound [35]. E-mail communication was found to be a convenient form of communication. Satisfaction of both patients and physicians improved in the e-mail group. The volume of messages and the time spent answering messages for the e-mail group of physicians did not increase. E-mail has the potential to improve the doctor-patient relationship as a result of better communication [36]. We hope that in the near future this consultation system will become more natural and familiar by using virtual environments too.

3.2. VR as a rehabilitation tool for the patients

VE and VR can be viewed as an advanced computer interface that allows the user to interact and become immersed within computer-generated simulated environments. Rapid development in modern technology and sophisticated computer systems have made it possible to display complex visual images that change in response to instructions from users on desktop computers. According to Lam et al. [37], the VEs demonstrate many of the characteristics of an ideal training medium. The VEs are especially valuable when training in real life situations would be impractical, dangerous, logistically difficult, unduly expensive or too difficult to control. The person can actively interact with simulated worlds by using interface devices. Its realism and versatility makes VR a suitable and innovative approach in rehabilitation. A number of researches have supported the use of VR in rehabilitation, in both assessment and treatment of physical, cognitive and psychological conditions [37].

The development work so far [38] has focused extensively and necessarily on the means to interface with the VE. In this phase we had to concentrate more upon the VE itself and how the system would be used as a rehabilitation tool in clinical practice. This required paying attention to the reasons why these types of technologies have potential value in rehabilitation, and why they might fail. The potential rehabilitation benefits of practice in a VE include: [38]

- Treatment of the cognitive process of task performance can take place more quickly in a VE than in a real environment.
- VE can avoid training in potentially hazardous settings.

- Working with VE can be enjoyable and compulsive, so providing motivational benefits.
- VE can allow the learning process to be more strictly controlled and defined than might be possible in the real environment.

The potential rehabilitation drawbacks of VEs are:

- Interfacing with the VE could be too difficult for patients to use. Patients cannot benefit from rehabilitation if they do not participate in it.
- The system could be too difficult, unrealistic or non-intuitive to be enjoyable and motivational. Patients may not benefit if not motivated.
- The system could fail to train the cognitive skills that are lost.
- Training in the virtual environment could fail if one has to generalise to real world settings.

In the following sections we give some examples of how VEs can be used in rehabilitation.

3.2.1. Haptic inferfacen

A haptic inferface was used for providing force feedback and a computer screen for the visual presentation of the virtual environment – the labyrinth. The rehabilitation training in the simple VE had a positive effect on the functional state of the patient's upper limbs [39]. The aim of another research project, the Gentle/S project, was to design and test a system that delivers interactive, robot mediated therapy for the upper limb (of stroke patients) [40].

GRAB is the name of a new Haptic and Audio Virtual Environment, which integrates a novel two-point force feedback device with a haptic audio geometric modeller. It was successfully tested by 52 visually impaired participants in a simple game [41].

Violin is a Multi-Mode browse, composed of three parts: 1. A vocal interpreter that handles communication with the user, 2. An agent, which downloads from the Internet the page requested by the user, 3. An agent which analyses the downloaded page and transforms it into vocal format in a way that can be browsed and navigated with the VoiceServer interpreter. Simsit is a Vocal Navigation in 3D Environments. Both Violin and SimSit were tested by students and children too [42].

A pen tablet based VR therapy tool for children with learning difficulties was developed in Japan. It aims to stimulate visual, audio and haptic sensation. It could be help for sensory integration and cognition treatment. It helped quantitative therapy and evaluation. The experiment was carried out with normal healthy children and confirmed the basic functions of this tool. [43]. In Japan a virtual 3D acoustic environment was created in which listeners feel a car passing in front of them to help them to learn to cross the street safely [44]. This system is useful not only for analyzing critical cues of perception of "crossablity" but also for training the blind how to cross a street.

3.2.2. Virtual environments for assessment

VR technology offers new options for neuropsychological assessment and cognitive rehabilitation. Empirical studies demonstrate its effectiveness. During the course of a collaborative VR research program at the University of Southern California and the Kessler Medical Rehabilitation Research and Education Corporation new VEs to help the attention process in children with ADHD within an HMD virtual classroom and the memory process in persons with TBI within a HMD virtual office [45, 46] were developed and evaluated.

Numerous studies using VEs have demonstrated that spatial knowledge can be effectively acquired from virtual exploration alone, and that such information can be readily transferred to real equivalent environments [47]. The test showed that the reaction time of groups who used VE significantly reduced [48].

Injuries related to falls are a major threat to the health of older people . A fall may not only result in an injury, but also in a decreased sense of autonomy in that person's daily life. In order to be able to prevent such falls it is necessary to understand the complex mechanisms involved in balance and walking. An immersive VR system was developed in which a person can move around, while being subjected to various events, which may influence balance and walking [49].

3.2.3. Speech, communication and acoustic virtual environment

VR is a useful tool for helping the communication of speech impaired persons. The various sign languages can be well animated in VE [50]. Tarnanas and Kikis conducted research comparing auditory feedback to visual and purely kinaesthetic feedback to find the most consistent feedback type that leads to developments in kinaesthesia, motor planning, sequencing and timing capabilities. Their results indicate that auditory feedback seems to be the most consistent type of feedback [51].

A practical implementation of various visual media, VR and associated technologies were developed as a therapy for special needs and rehabilitation [52]. The results show that immersion in a VE can hold similar potential to immersion in an audible environment for such children. The attraction and advantages of using neither wearable nor tactile sensors but merely exploiting the unencumbered movement of the children through space was readily apparent. It was also apparent that when the individual feedback was singular, certain users were more perceptive to audio while others were more perceptive to visual stimuli [52].

One important application of VR is to train blind users to navigate and move around in real environment. A spatial audio system was designed for blind users by Kurniawan and co-workers. This system was able to simulate the sound variation in different room sizes successfully [53].

3.2.4. Stroke rehabilitation

Many applications have been developed all over the world for stroke rehabilitation. One of the most interesting of these researches is the VividGroup's Gesture Xtreme System [54, 55]. It is a unique approach to VR, which might have important applications for the rehabilitation of children and adults with physical and/or cognitive impairment (www.vividgroup.com). Another way to develop VR applications is to start from existing occupational treatment methods and to develop platforms for home rehabilitation. Such telemedically controlled systems using low-cost web-based video/audio telemedicine units have high much potential [56]. Connor et al. in San Francisco used a haptic guided error-free learning unit with an active force feedback joystick and computer for rehabilitation of cognitive deficits following a stroke [57].

To test spatial memory a virtual reality Arena task was designed, consisting of a circular space surrounded by pattern rendered walls. The participants had to navigate within the arena using a joystick to signal motion. Brain activity was recorded during the different phases of the task in control participants and then in patients who have damage to the hippocampus [58].

The project called "Virtual Reality for Brain Injury Rehabilitation" developed at Lund University in Sweden produced many interesting results. They investigated usability issues of VR technology for people with brain injury, examined the issue of transfer and training, developed different applications of VR for training in daily tasks, such as kitchen work, using an automatic teller machine, finding one's way in a complex environment, using virtual vending and automatic service machines [59, 60]. VR has been used to test executive functioning in patients with focal frontal lesions. It was carried out in a multi-componential VR procedure, the Bungalow Task, and was developed to test strategy formation, rule breaking and prospective memory [61].

The V.E.Ne.Re. (Virtual Executive NEuropsychologocal Rehabilitation) consists in the construction and validation of artificial environments based on VR technologies, aimed at the cognitive rehabilitation of executive functions (frontal lobe dysfunction; dysexecutive syndrome) [62].

A new VE was studied to examine the possibility to influence empathy on caregiver personnel. The VE looked like a normal apartment and could be experienced with or without different perceptual disorders of stroke. Results from observations and interviews indicate that the simulator, in spite of problems of usability, was effective in influencing caregivers empathy [63].

3.2.5. Virtual travel training

Childhood development is directly related to being able to independently explore, manoeuvre and interact with one's environment. A Virtual Environment Mobility Simulator was developed in Ireland to provide a simple and cost effective choice for powered wheelchair training and rehabilitation [64].

Brown et al. have produced a flexible travel training environment to support constructive training for people with learning disabilities [65]. In another study for training of people with learning disability to travel independently showed how the skills learned in the VE appeared to transfer to the real world [66]. Lam e al. carried out a pilot study to develop street survival skills of people who had had a stroke using a 2D interactive VR program [37]. The results of the training in a non immersive interactive VE showed improvement in the ability of patients who suffered from Unilateral Spatial Neglect (as a result of a right hemisphere stroke) to cross a real street [67].

To many people, the ability to drive is an important aspect of their life and a symbol of their independence. However, after brain injury, or approaching old age, although people often feel that they are able to resume or continue driving, they are not always safe to do so. In the University of East London a VR-based driving assessment was designed which allows people to test their driving ability off-road and thereby help them to come to a more informed decision as to whether they should resume driving or continue to drive [68].

3.2.6. VR for special needs

Leonard and co-workers used the Single-User Virtual Environment of a café to test how seven teenagers with an Autistic Spectrum Disorder could cope with finding a place to sit in differing situations [69]. This study has shown the potential for teaching and learning social skills in this "safe" and calm alternative to in situ social skills training locations.

The game project by Swedish Library of Talking Books and Braille showed that it is possible to create fun computer games for partially sighthed or blind children. In sound based games, the player obtains a mental image of all objects and characters that are present by listening to the sounds with which they are associated. [70].

Three pilot studies were carried out in order to investigate the EyeToy's (www.EyeToy.com) potential for use in the rehabilitation of people who are elderly and have disabilities [71]. Terraformers (www.terraformers.nu) is the result of three years practical research in developing a real-time 3D graphic game accessible to blind and low vision players as well as full sighted players. The idea was to try to bridge the gap in the game industry between the mass market 3D games for full sighted and the sound only games for blind and low vision players [72]. This game won the "Innovation in Audio Award at the 2003 Independent Games Festival (www.igf.com).

For us one of the most interesting application of VE was the interactive painting [73] where, through utilizing computer technology and human machine interfaces (sensors and cameras) to stimulate complementary senses, visual and tactile interpretation of music was enabled giving new meaning and understanding to handicapped people. The Soundbeam is a mature and sophisticated ultrasound movement sensor that detects movement along its linear axis. It translates movement to MIDI [73].

3.2.7. Virtual reality therapy for anxiety disorders

Brenda K. and Mark D. Wiederhold wrote an excellent book on the topic of Virtual Reality therapy for anxiety disorders [74], therefore we will not discuss this question. The reader can find everything about treatment of panic disorders, agoraphobia, posttraumatic stress disorders, specific pho-bias and social phobia, aviophobia, fear of driving, acrophobia, claustro-phobia, arachnophobia and fear of medical procedures using VR in this recent book.

3.2.8. Painkilling with VR

A special use of VR is in pain relief. VR treatment is being used as a distraction technique to reduce pain associated with wound care in burn victims [74]. Hoffman et al. explored the use of "SpiderWorld", originally created to treat those with arachnophobia, which included a kitchen with virtual objects and cabinet doors that could be opened and closed on two patients [75]. In a second study Hoffmann used VR distraction for 12 patients with burns during physical therapy procedures [74, 75]. In another study participants were placed in either a "low technology VR condition", or a "high technology VR condition", or into a control condition with no VR. As the research predicted, those in the "high tech" condition reported less pain and reported feeling more "present" in the virtual world [74, 75].

3.3. Virtual humans

For a better 'human' feeling avatars are used in VEs. Nowadays the expectations are that avatars should look more and more like the real human body and face with emotions.

A new avatar was developed in Greece using VRML to produce the exact gestures represented in the sign language notation [76].

A set of immersive CyberTherapy applications was implemented using a high performance portable virtual reality platform, called the Virtual Human Interface (VHI) [77, 78]. The VHI was specifically developed to place the users into closed loop VE in which they face a variety of challenges to help them gradually overcome their respective disorders in a fast and effective manner. To support this functionality the VHI system not only presents complex, photo-realistic stimuli to its users but also measures reactions and employs biofeedback to keep the patient constantly at his or her maximal tolerance level as part of the interaction process (Fig 1). In addition another unique feature of the VHI is its ability to create and animate high fidelity digital humans capable of expressing subtle facial expressions and nonverbal signals or body language. These virtual humans are seamlessly integrated with CyberTherapy applications opening a new avenue and building a solid foundation for future research.

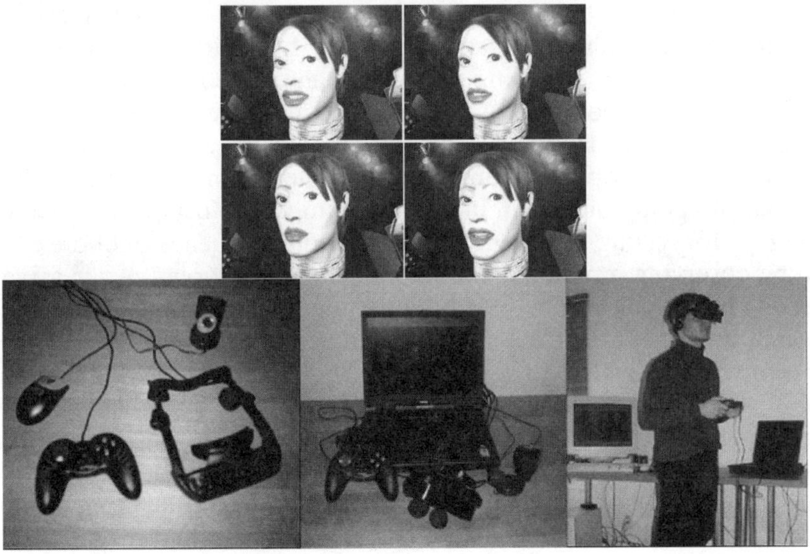

Fig 1. Digital Face and the VR System

3.4. Is Virtual reality dangerous for young children?

Play is essential for children's learning. Toys are the tools of play. Which games are provided and how they are used are equally important. Parents often ask their paediatrician for advice about appropriate toys, books, computer or video games, because they know that these tools may be im-portant in their child's development. When paediatricians advise parents, it is important to stress that toys serve a supportive role in enhancing a child's development. Play materials should match the developmental and individual needs of each child. Some children may need toys that have been adapted to accommodate a motor, visual, or other disability. All chil-dren benefit from toys that promote safe physical activity [79]. How do we stand in relation to the intellectual and spiritual growth of young children? We need to be more concerned than ever about the suitability of real-life news violence for children. Despite the evident importance of teaching children to become critical viewers of violence in entertainment programs, health care professionals and parents also need to emphasize the potentially negative effects of real violence portrayed in news programs [80]. An anonymous self-report assisted survey was administered to an opportunistic sample of parents/guardians who visited child health providers at 3 sites: an urban children's hospital clinic, an urban managed care clinic, and a suburban private practice in January 1999 to July 2000. The parent questionnaire included questions on child-rearing attitudes and practices and sociodemographic information. Among children who watched television, parents reported that they spent an average of 2.6 hours per day watching television. Twenty-eight percent of parents stated that their youngest child played an average of 1.6 hours per day with video games (median: 1.0 hours). Preschool children spent the most time watching television and videos and playing video games. After preschool, there was a decrease in the number of hours per day watching television and videos but not in video game play [81]. Video games are increasingly becoming a part of entertainment, virtual reality applications are going on sale in increasing numbers. Most of these games are dangerous for young children, because media influences children - they learn by observing, imitating, and internalising behaviours. Aggressive attitudes and behaviours are learned by imitating observed models [82, 83, 84]. Research has shown that the strongest single correlate with violent behaviour is previous exposure to violence [85, 86, 87]. Because children younger than 8 years cannot discriminate between fantasy and reality, they are uniquely vulnerable to learning and adopting as reality the circumstances, attitudes, and behaviours portrayed by entertainment media [88, 89, 90, 91]. The early home environment, including cognitive stimulation, emotional support, and exposure to television, has a significant impact on bullying in grade school [92]. Maybe these children need virtual reality rehabilitation in the future to compensate for earlier influence of virtual reality worlds. The main problem is: although the entertainment industry currently sees little problem with the quality of their product, the research literature and most parents would disagree. American media are the most graphically violent and sexually suggestive in the world. At present, networks, studios, and software companies have little incentive to create more educational and healthier programming [93].

4. Medical informatics VR research in Hungary and the developed VEs

After reviewing the medical use of VR we would like to give an the example from our laboratory of how educational VR programs can be developed effectively in a university environment. Multimedia and Virtual Reality have been subject choices for informatics engineer students since 1998 and 1999 at our University. The courses consist of two lecture hours and three practice hours per week. In the practice classes the students learn the use of Macromedia Director, Flash, Maya and VRML. They have to prepare software, objects and virtual environments for the research work going on in the Colour and Multimedia Laboratory of the Faculty of Technical Informatics at the University of Veszprém. More then 40 software packages were developed for rehabilitation in the past ten years in our laboratory. These software packages are used not only in Hungary but abroad too. The following chapters give some examples.

Phobia treatment: The aim of our work at the University of Veszprém and SOTE (Semmelweis Medical University in Budapest) was to create VE, which could be used in treating phobias. Of course we were unable to deal with all of the existing phobias, we created virtual worlds for treating agoraphobia (fear of wide, open spaces), acrophobia (fear of height) and specific phobia (fear of traveling). Our investigations were the first in Hungary.

The first environment is a simple balcony of a two-storey house. It has a large tiled floor and low fence all around it. In the initial scene we can see the top of some trees and some houses (Fig 2). After starting the animation the viewpoint takes the users closer and closer to the fence and makes them look down to the garden [94].

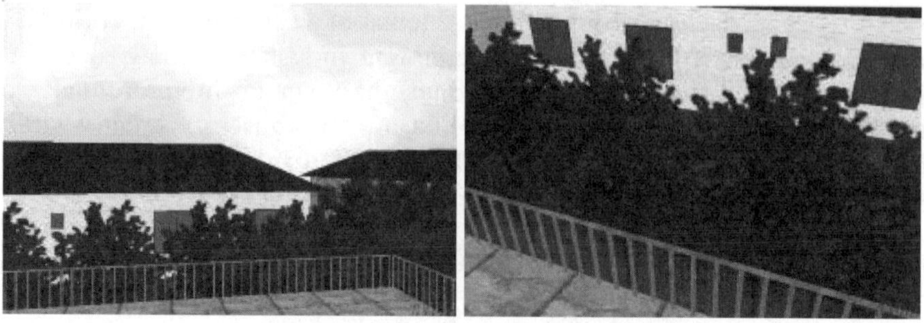

Fig 2. Virtual balcony: the initial scene and looking down.

Another program to treat acrophobia is an external glass elevator environment. It shows a ten-storey high building with an external glass elevator. At the beginning the elevator is on the ground floor (Fig 3). Then the elevator starts up and finally one has the view from the top of the building. These VEs were created by the help of VRML.

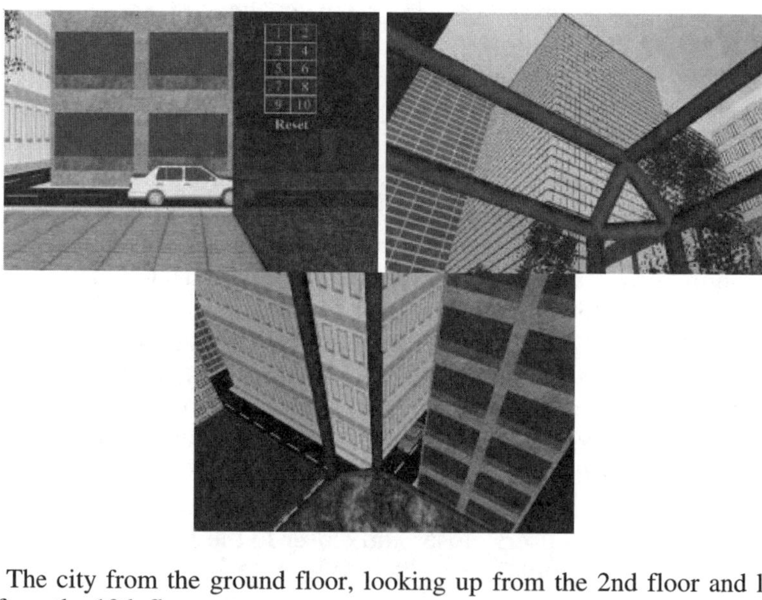

Fig 3. The city from the ground floor, looking up from the 2nd floor and looking down from the 10th floor.

The internal glass elevator is very similar to the external one, but there are some differences. The main difference is that we developed this virtual environment by using the program Maya. The main reason for using another method for development was to compare the development environments.

First we made actual video recordings in a hotel in Budapest. The model of the internal glass elevator was based on the real pictures from these video recordings. We wanted to compare not only the development environments (VRML and Maya) but also the virtual worlds (Fig 4 and Fig 5) with real video recording in treating phobias.

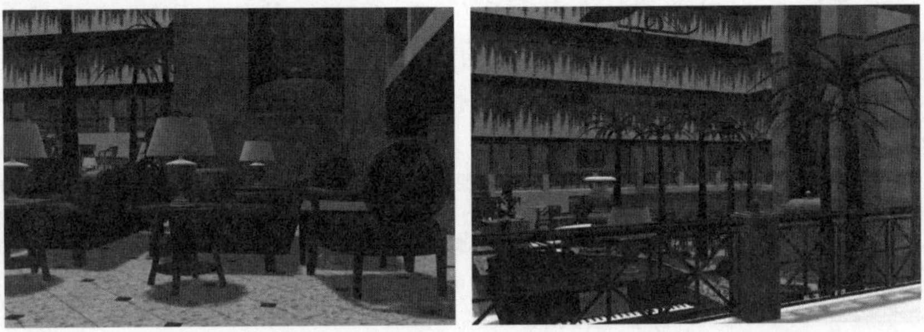

Fig 4. Entering into the virtual hotel and view from the first floor.

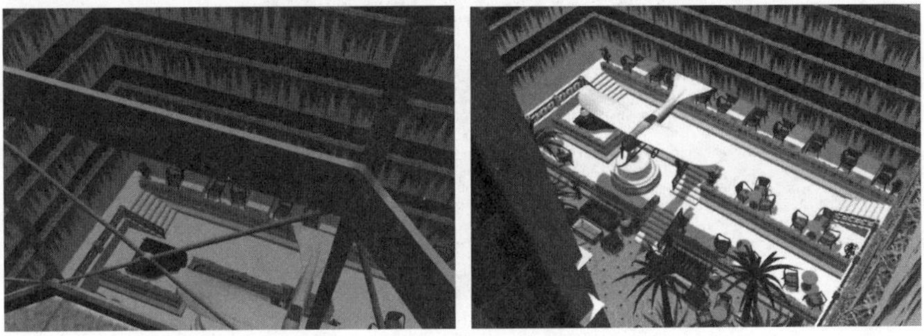

Fig 5. View from the glass elevator and from the 10th floor.

For specific phobias (fear of travelling) we modelled underground travelling in Budapest. (Fig 6 and Fig 7) [95]. First we prepared videos of this underground and then based on these videos we created the virtual underground with the help of Maya software. After modelling the underground with Maya we exported the virtual objects to Shockwave 3D file format (the extension of this file is W3D). We had to do this to make the VE interactive. For exporting we used Shockwave Exporter that could be found free on the Web. This program is able to export Maya made objects to the (W3D) format that can easily be used by Multimedia Director.

For the VE we cut the sounds from the real video to increase the feeling of reality. These sounds were applied to the prepared virtual world. The voices increase the sensation that the patients feel like being on the escalator or getting on a platform. Some special sound effects, for example the voice indicating the departure of the underground train, have particular part as the sufferer feels the same anxiety as he/she feels while travelling on real trains. It turned out that by adding sound the same feeling of reality could be evoked with less detailed images than without sound.

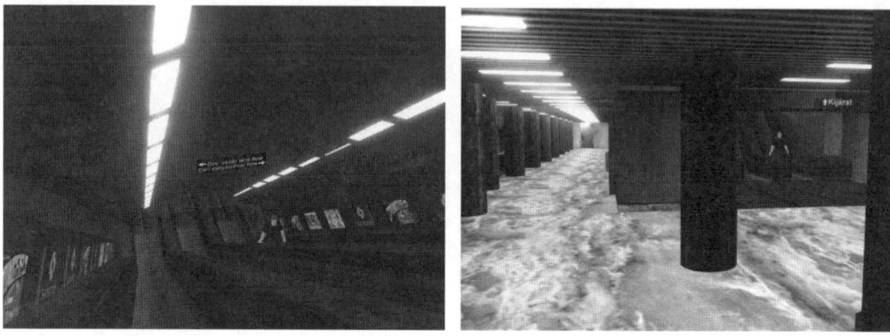

Fig 6. The escalator and the underground waiting hall.

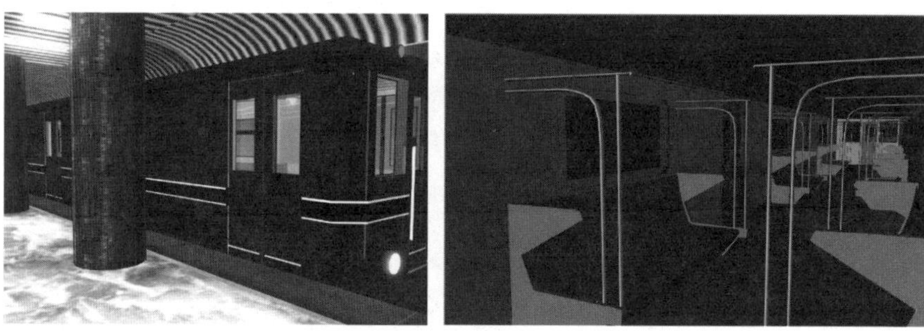

Fig 7. The underground carriages outside and inside.

We developed VE for claustrophobia too: a closed lift and a room, where the wall could be moved. We tested our VE by the help of the psychological institute of SOTE and some students, who suffered with mild phobias. The clinical test with the patients who suffered from severe, complex phobias began in the second half of 2005.

For the education of autistic children we developed a virtual shopping software. (Fig 8) This educational software was developed using Dark Basic programming language [96]. We are testing the virtual shopping scenario in a special school for children with learning difficulties in Veszprém. The Virtual Shop project builds on their visual perception, applying symbol-cards and an audio-visual virtual environment. On the lower left corner of Fig 8. The user can see a shopping list. The shopping is easier for the child if he/she can use this list and the symbol cards. The actual item of the shopping list is not only shown but is also spoken. The goal of preparing the software was to produce a useful support for education. The application is designed to be used in the teaching process or even at home - with the help of someone to monitor - as a playful way of learning. Based on the advice of teachers educating autistic children, the software uses speech to guide the user in combination with visual support, with the aim of improving verbal comprehension and communication.

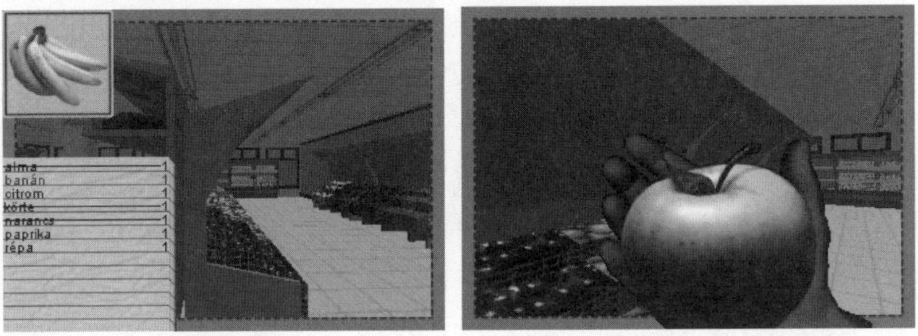

Fig 8. The virtual shopping.

Our newest project has been prepared in cooperation with the National Centre of Brain Vein Diseases, Budapest developing a virtual home for aphasic patients. The aim of our work here was to teach everyday words to stroke patients [97].

An average family house and its equipments provides the most suitable environment for the cognitive treatment of aphasic stroke patients. The ideal situation would be to develop for every patient his or her own house. The patients could most easily develop their skills in this virtual environment. The patients could identify the objects in their familiar environment and would develop proper orientation in that environment. But it is an impossible task to develop for everybody their own virtual home. Development of a virtual home is a considerable job and requires a lot of time. Therefore we paid a lot of attention to choosing the model of the house. We chose an average blueprint of houses built in Hungary.

Selecting a large enough floor-place was the most important initial decision, because we needed enough room for movement in the house. The first essential task was modelling the kitchen. The most important household equipment and objects for everyday life are found here and there are many objects that have a potential for causing accidents. The user can find there ordinary kitchen equipment, for example the microwave oven, the fridge, the gas-cooker and so on. There are some possibilities to extend the number of equipment, objects, and of course the house.

In the design phase we had to take into account that we were developing a virtual environment for aphasic patients. This produced some special tasks, for example we have not modelled a very modern and futuristic house, because an unreal virtual environment would not have been acceptable to our patients.

One of the most important expectations of the virtual house is that it contains a lot of objects. The patient's task at this rehabilitation phase is to name more and more objects. Increasing the number of objects increases the number of tasks too. The objects modelled are typical objects that every patient has met in their life. The everyday objects are, for example, a cup, a plate and a knife. We modelled the objects in such a form that their shapes are very simple and ordinary.

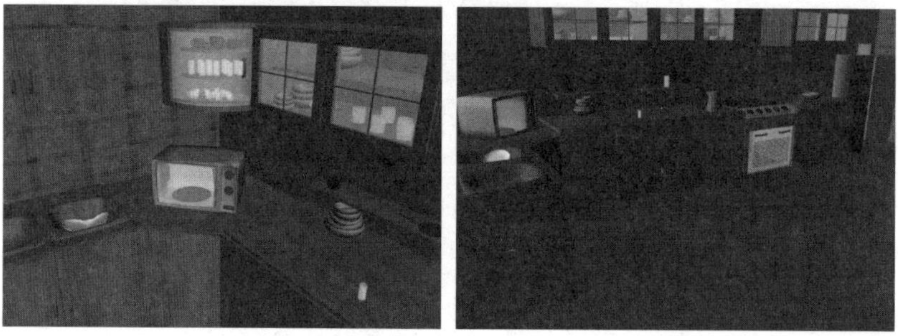

Fig 9. The kitchen in the virtual home

The tasks in the virtual home are:

- To name the object: The patient has to name the objects when the therapists points to them.
- To find one place in the building: The patient has to learn to orient himself in the house. For example he or she has to find the way to the kitchen from a pre-defined place set by the doctor.
- To find the objects in the building by their name: This is already a very complex task. For example the patient has to find the cup. The patient has to know where he or she is, in which direction to start and where the cup might be found. If the patient reaches the correct location he or she has to identify the cup.
- To find objects that do not fit into the environment: The essence of the task is that an object had been placed in a location in the house that is not normal for the given object. For example a pan-cake grill has been placed in the drawing room. The patient has to recognize that this is not a usual place for the grill and has to tell its name.
- Checking the route: The therapist investigates how easily the patients get from one place to the other, how well they orient themselves.

- To practise everyday tasks: The patients are given the possibility of performing everyday tasks, for example, laying a table or deciding on the order of different tasks.

We hope that the virtual world can be used for patients with mild and relatively mild brain damage. The testing of the virtual world will start next year.

We hope that these examples demonstrate what, even in a small university group, students can learn the design of VEs by preparing useful programs for rehabilitation, rather than everyday shooting games.

5. Future

Augmented reality might be one future direction. Some computer games were developed by the MindGames team in Media Lab Europe. These games share the central concern of helping the users learn constructive skills, such as relaxation, attention and deep breathing that can have physical and mental benefits in their everyday lives. This involves augmenting the traditional methods of biofeedback with sensory immersion, novel signal processing, compelling game play within the context of an "intelligent" computer system that receives feedback from the person and learns to alter the environment according to its emotional state [98].

The main disadvantage of a current immersive VR system, like a CAVE is its high cost, high complexity and inability to be applied in a multi-user environment. In addition, these complex tools cannot be operated on the Internet. With rapid improvements in computers and network, new inexpensive VR technologies are being developed and one of them is called virtual reality modelling language (VRML). VRML runs on a personal computer and can be operated on the Internet easily. Researchers are also developing some easily used toolkits for visualization. The purpose of this research and development work is to employ common VR and visualization tools for implementing VRLE and to try to share experience with others who have developed similar system without a professional knowledge of VR or techniques.

Augmenting the VR programs with devices such as data gloves is still expensive, but with the evolution of the VR game industry more and more new equipment will be on the market and will hopefully become cheaper. In this case the "old" but usable PC-s and game hardware could be used at home or in the clinic for rehabilitation of disabled people. VR researchers are investigating the possibility of delivering VE over the Internet. Eventually it will be possible to offer VR services to patients under the supervision of special teachers, doctors or therapists in their homes. In this case the patient and the therapist could go into the same VE at the same time, or hopefully in the near future more patients could work collaboratively with their therapist in the same VE at the same time.

6. Conclusion

While interest in the medical informatics discipline is growing, the number of core contributors to VR research remains relatively small. Two major questions for the discipline are: What are the research challenges that informatics faces today? How can the discipline be strengthened and positioned to maximize its success in addressing those challenges? Progress toward research challenges formulated more than ten years ago has been varied. While many new technologies have become available for clinical practice, research, and education, many fundamental problems remain to be addressed by informatics research. Recommendations to augment the research capacity in informatics include creating a stronger worldwide informatics research community and drawing more biomedical informatics-, psychologist- and clinical staff researchers to VR research areas.

We hope that the number of investigations conducted in the field of VR for medical informatics and rehabilitation will grow. Computer graphics are better now and the 3D rendering techniques are becoming more mature, thus contributing to the reality.

The review of current VR applications shows that VR can be considered a useful tool for diagnosis, education and training of healthcare staff and also an education, training and rehabilitation tool for patients. We hope VR will be a new and useful tool for distance learning, distributed training and e-therapy. If we take into consideration that nowadays young active people (less than 30 years old) grow up with computer games and VR technology we can be sure that for them it would be natural to use the same equipment and IT tools in their rehabilitation 30 or 40 years from now. VR will already be a part of their natural everyday real environment.

But there are some critical questions too. What is the situation with the youngest children? Is VR really dangerous for them? Where is the limit to the use of VR? Are there any ethical standards? These questions are still open. We can only hope that the scientists and users will find the optimal use of this new technology and will not use it for virtual ' killings' as in many games now on the market.

References

1. Bowman, D.A., Kruijff, E., LaViola Jr., J.J., I Poupyrev, I., 3D User Interfaces. Addison-Wesley, 2004, pp. 7.
2. Stanney, K.M., Handbokk of virtual environments, In: Stanney, K.M. editor, Handbook of Virtual Environments: Design, Implementation and Applications. Mahwah, N.J.: Lawrence Erlbaum Associates, Inc.; 2002, pp. 301-302.
3. Rosenberg H, Grad HA, Matear DW, The effectiveness of computer-aided, self-instructional programs in dental education: a systematic review of the literature, in J Dent Educ 2003;67:524–532.
4. Brusilovsky, P., Methods and techniques of adaptive hypermedia, in User Modeling and User-Adapted Interaction 1996;6:87–129
5. Corbett, A.T., Koedinger, K.R., Anderson, J.R., Intelligent tutoring systems. In: Handbook of human-computer interaction. Helander MG, Landauer TK, Prabhu PV, editors. Amsterdam: Elsevier Science BV., 1997, pp. 849–874.
6. Johnson, L.A., Cunningham,M.A., Finkelstein, M.W., Hand, J.S., Geriatric patient simulations for dental hygiene, in J Dent Educ 1997;61:667–677.
7. Dev, P., Montgomery, K., Senger, S., Heinrichs, W.L., Srivastava, S., Waldron, K., Simulated Medical Learning Environments on the Internet, in J. Am. Med. Inform. Assoc. 2002;9(5):437-447
8. Tsai, M.C., Godin, P.J., Melmon, K.L., Dev, P., Wood, W.H., Hubbs, P.R., et al., Integrating information for medical decision support and education: a model for other knowledge domains, Brighton, UK: Second International and Interdisciplinary Workshop: Intelligent Information Integration, 13th Biennial European Conference on Artificial Intelligence (ECAI-98).
9. Dornan T, Maredia N, Hosie L, et al. A web-based presentation of an undergraduate clinical skills curriculum. Medical Education 2003;37(6):500-8.
10. Hoffmann, H., Murray, M., Curlee, R., Fritchle, A., Anatomic visualizeR: teaching and learning anatomy with virtual reality. In: Akay M, Marsh A, editors. In formation technologies in medicine, Volume I: Medical Simulation and Education. New York: Willey; 2001.
11. Temkin, B., Acosta, E., Hatfield, P., Onal, E., Tong, A., Web-based Three-dimensional Virtual Body Structures: W3D-VBS, J. Am. Med. Inform. Assoc. 2002;9(5):425-436.
12. Walker, D.S., Lee, W.Y., Skov, N.M., Berger, C.F., Athley, B.D., Investigating Users' Requirements: Computer-based Anatomy Learning Modules for Multiple User Test Beds, J Am Med Inform Assoc 2002;9(4):311-319.
13. Lu, J., Pan, Z., Lin, H., Zhang, M., Shi, J., Virtual learning environment for medical education based on VRML and VTK. in Computers & Graphics, 2005;29(2):283-288
14. A Path From the National Library of Medicine?s AnatLine Database to 3D Virtual Reality Modeling Language Models, available: http://www.nlm.nih.gov/research/visible/vhpconf2000/AUTHORS/JOHNSON/MOVIINDX.HTM.
15. Wacholder, N., Imielinska, C., Johnson, S., Soliz, E. Molholt, P., Implications of 3D visualization for medical education, Stud Health Technol Inform, 1998;50: 377-8.

16. Stewart, J.E., Graham, R.S., Broaddus, W.C., Johnson, J.H. Hack, G.D., Improved 3D anatomic understanding through stereoscopic visualization, In: Banvard RA, Pinciroli F, Cerveri P, editors. 2nd Visible Human Project Conference Proceedings; 1998 Oct 1-2; Bethesda, CD-ROM
17. Rigamonti, D.D., Bryant, H.J., Bustos, O., Smirniotopoulos, J.G., Moore, L. Hoffman, H.M., Implementing Anatomic VisualizeR? learning modules in anatomy education, In: Banvard, R.A., editor. The Visible Human Project Conference Proceedings [CD-ROM]; 2000 Oct 5-6; Bethesda
18. Chiou, R.C.H., Kaufman, A.E., Liang, Z., Unified Analysis, Modeling, Matching and Synthesis for CT Color Texture Mapping From the Visible Human Data Set, available at: http://www.nlm.nih.gov/research/visible/vhpconf98/AUTHORS/CHIOU/CHIOU.HTM
19. Greenes R.A., Lorenzi, N.M., Audacious Goals for Health and Biomedical Informatics in the New Millennium, in J Am Med Inform Assoc 1998;5(5):395-400.
20. Handels, H., Ehrhardt, J., Plötz, W., Pöppl, S.J., Simulation of Hip Operations and Design of Custom-made Endoprostheses using Virtual Reality Techniques, in Methods of Information in Medicine, 2001;40(2):74-77
21. Mazziotta, J., Toga, A., Evans, A., at al., A Four-Dimensional Probabilistic Atlas of the Human Brain, J Am Med Inform Assoc 2001;8(5):401-430.
22. Chun, J., Kim, H., Lee, S.G., Choi, J., Cho, H., A DBMS-based Medical Teleconferencing System, J. Am. Med. Inform. Assoc., 2001; 8(5): 460 - 467.
23. Iskra, K.A., Belleman, R.G., van Albada, G.D., Santoso, J., Sloot, P.M.A., Bal, H.E., Spoelder, H.J.W., Bubak, M., The Polder Computing Environment: a system for interactive distributed simulation, Concurrency and Computation: Practice and Experience, 2002;14(13-15): 1313-1335.
24. Poliakov, A.V., Albright, E., Hinshaw, K.P., Corina, D.P., Ojemann, G., Martin, R.F., Brinkley, J.F., Server-based Approach to Web Visualization of Integrated Three-dimensional Brain Imaging Data, J. Am. Med. Inform. Assoc. 2005;12(2):140-151.
25. Leslie, L., Rappo, P., Abelson, H., Jenkins, R.R., Sewall, S.R., Chesney, R.W., Mulvey, H.J., Simon, J.L., Alden, E.R., Final Report of the FOPE II Pediatric Generalists of the Future Workgroup, Pediatrics, 2000; 106(5): 1199-1223.
26. Sung, W.H., Fung, C.P., Chen, A.C., Yuan, C.C., Ng. H.T., Doong, J.L., The assessment of stability and reliability of a virtual reality-based laporoscopic gynecology simulation system. Eur J Gynaecol Oncol 2003;24(2):143-6
27. Friedl, R., Preisack, M.B., Klas, W. Rose, T., Stracke, S., Quast, K.J., at al. Virtual Reality and 3D Visualizations in Heart Surgery Education, Heart Surg Forum, 2002;5(3):e17-21.
28. Gor, M., McCloy, R., Stone R., Smith, A., Virtual reality laparoscopic simulator for assessment in gynaecology. Bjog, 2003;110(2):181-7.
29. Herfarth, C., Lamade W., Fisher L., Chiu, P., Cardenas, C., Thorn., M., et al. The effect of virtual reality training on liver operation planning. Swiss Surg, 2002;8(2):67-73.
30. Satava, R.M., Jones, S.B., Medical appliacations of virtual reality. In: Stanney, K.M. editor, Handbook of Virtual Environments: Design, Implementation and

Applications. Mahwah, N.J.: Lawrence Erlbaum Associates, Inc.; 2002. pp. 368-391.

31. Moorthy, K., Smith, S., Brown, T., Bann, S., Darzi, A., Evaluation of virtual reality bronhoscopy as a learning and assessment tool. Respiration 2003;70(2):195-9.
32. Dunkin, B.J., Flexible endoscope simulators. Semin Laparosc Surg, 2003;10(1):29-35.
33. Robb, R.A., Virtual (Computed) Endoscopy, available: http://www.nlm.nih.gov/ research/visible/vhp_conf/robb/robb_pap.htm
34. Riva, G., Applications of Virtual Environmnets in medicine, Methods of Information in Medicine, 2003;42(5):524-534.
35. Kedar, i., Ternullo, J.L., Weinrib, C.E., Kelleher, K.M., Brandling-Bennett, H., Kvedar, J.C., Internet based consultations to transfer knowledge for patients requiring specialised care, BMJ, 2003; 326(7391):696-699. available at: The general medical journal website http://bmj.bmjjournals.com/
36. Leong, S.J., Gingrich, D., Lewis, P.R., Mauger, D.T., George, J.H., Enhancing Doctor-Patient Communication Using Email: A Pilot Study, J. Am. Board Fam. Pract., 2005; 18(3): 180 - 188.
37. Lam, Y.S., Tam, S.F., Man, D.W.K., Weis, P.L., Evaluation of a computer assisted 2D interactive virtual reality system in training street survival skills of people with stroke. Proc. 5th Intl Conf. on Disability, Virtual Reality and Assoc. Technologies, in Sharkey, McRindle &Brown (Eds), pp. 27-32, Oxford, UK, 20-22 Sept. 2004.
38. Edmans, J.A., Gladman, J., Walker, M., Sunderland, A., Porter, A., Stanton Fraser, D., Mixed reality environments in stroke rehabilitation: development as rehabilitation tools. in the Proc. of The 5th International Conference on Disability, Virtual Reality and Associated Technologies, Oxford, UK, 20-22 Sept., 2004, pp. 3-10.
39. Bardorfer, A., Munih, M., Zupan, A., Primožič, A., Rehabilitation Training in Virtual Environment Using Haptic interface – Case Study, Assistive Technologies – Added Value to the Quality of Life, Ĉ. Marinĉek et al. (Eds.) IOS Press, 2001, pp.251-255.
40. van de Hel, P.K.M., Driessen, B.J.F., Oderwald, M.P., Gentle/S: Robot mediated therapy for stroke patients in a virtual world makes exercising more enjoyable and effective, Assistive Technologies – Added Value to the Quality of Life, Ĉ. Marinĉek et al. (Eds.) IOS Press, 2001, pp.255-261.
41. Maggennis, M., Gallagher, B., Wood, J., Arias, E.C., Sevilla, J.M., Gladsote, K., Graupp, H., Gutierrez, T., Avizzano, C., Bergamasco, M., GRAB – A new haptic and audio virtual environment enabling vision impaired people to access the three-dimensional computer graphic world. Assistive Technologies – Shaping the Future, G.M. Craddock et al. (Eds.) IOS Press, 2003, pp.471-475.
42. Barbieri, T., Sbattella, L., Virtual Sounds and Virtual Spaces to support Persons with Cognitive and Physical Disabilities during Information Retrieval, Rehabilitation and Learning, Assistive Technologies – Shaping the Future, G.M. Craddock et al. (Eds.) IOS Press, 2003, pp.1011-1015.

43. Takahashi, Y., Ito, Y., Yamashita, T., Terada, T., Inoue, K., Ikeda, Y., Suzuki, K., Lee, H., Komeda, T., Virtual Reality Based Therapy Application for Developmental Disordered Children, Computers Helping People with Special Needs, K. Miesenberger at al. (Eds.) Springer Press, 2004, pp. 369-376.
44. Shiosie, T., Ito, K., Mamada, K., The Development of Virtual 3D Acoustic Environment for Training "Perception of Crossability", Computers Helping People with Special Needs, K. Miesenberger at al. (Eds.) Springer Press, 2004, pp. 476-483.
45. Rizzo, A.A., Bowerly, T., Buckwalter, J.G., Schultheis, M., Matheis, R., Shahabi, C., Neumann, U., Kim, L., Sharifzadeh, M., Virtual environments for the assessment of attention and memory process: the virtual classroom and office. Proc. 4th Intl Conf. on Disability, Virtual Reality and Assoc. Technologies, in Sharkey, Sik Lányi & Standen (Eds.) pp. 3-12, Veszprém, Hungary, 18-20 Sept. 2002.
46. Rizzo, A.A., Pryor, L., Matheis, R., Schulteis, M., Ghahremani, K., Sey, A., Memory assesement using graphics-based and panoramic video virtual environments. Proc. 5th Intl Conf. on Disability, Virtual Reality and Assoc. Technologies, in Sharkey, McRindle &Brown (Eds), pp. 331-338, Oxford, UK, 20-22 Sept. 2004.
47. Stanton, D., Foreman, N., Wilson, P., Duffi, H., Parnell, R., Use of virtual environments to acquire understanding of real-world multi-level environments. Proc. 4th Intl Conf. on Disability, Virtual Reality and Assoc. Technologies, in Sharkey, Sik Lányi & Standen (Eds.) pp. 13-18, Veszprém, Hungary, 18-20 Sept. 2002.
48. Standen, P.J., Ip, W.M.D., An evaluation of the use of virtual environments in improving choice reaction time in people with severe intellectual disabilities. Proc. 4th Intl Conf. on Disability, Virtual Reality and Assoc. Technologies, in Sharkey, Sik Lányi & Standen (Eds.) pp. 19-24, Veszprém, Hungary, 18-20 Sept. 2002.
49. Nyberg, L., Lundin-Olsson, L., Sondell, B., Backman, A., Holmlund, K., Eriksson, S., Stenvall M., Rosendahl, E., Maxhall, M., Bucht, G., Development of a virtual reality system to study tendency of falling among older people. Proc. 5th Intl Conf. on Disability, Virtual Reality and Assoc. Technologies, in Sharkey, McRindle &Brown (Eds), pp. 315-320, Oxford, UK, 20-22 Sept. 2004.
50. Murakami, M., Kuroda, T., Manabe, Y., Chihara, K., Generation of modifier representation in sign animation. Proc. 4th Intl Conf. on Disability, Virtual Reality and Assoc. Technologies, in Sharkey, Sik Lányi & Standen (Eds.) pp. 27-32, Veszprém, Hungary, 18-20 Sept. 2002.
51. Tarnanas, I., Kikis, V., Sound-kinetic feedback for virtual therapeutic environments. Proc. 4th Intl Conf. on Disability, Virtual Reality and Assoc. Technologies, in Sharkey, Sik Lányi & Standen (Eds.) pp. 191-196, Veszprém, Hungary, 18-20 Sept. 2002.
52. Brooks, T., Camurri, A., Canagarajah, N., Hasselblad, S., Interaction with shapes and sounds as a therapy for special needs and rehabilitation. Proc. 4th Intl Conf. on Disability, Virtual Reality and Assoc. Technologies, in Sharkey,

Sik Lányi & Standen (Eds.) pp. 205-212, Veszprém, Hungary, 18-20 Sept. 2002.

53. Kurniawan, S.H., Sporka, A., Nemec, V., Slavik, P., Design and user evaluation of a spatial audio system for blind users. Proc. 5th Intl Conf. on Disability, Virtual Reality and Assoc. Technologies, in Sharkey, McRindle &Brown (Eds), pp. 175-182, Oxford, UK, 20-22 Sept. 2004.
54. Kizony, R., Katz, N., Weingarden, H., Weiss, P.L., Immersion without encumbrance: adapting a virtual reality system for the rehabilitation of individuals with stroke and spinal cord injury. Proc. 4th Intl Conf. on Disability, Virtual Reality and Assoc. Technologies, in Sharkey, Sik Lányi & Standen (Eds.) pp. 55-62, Veszprém, Hungary, 18-20 Sept. 2002.
55. Kizony, R., Katz, N., Weiss, P.L., Virtual reality based intervention in rehabilitation: relationship between motor and cognitive abilities and performance within virtual environments for patients with stroke. Proc. 5th Intl Conf. on Disability, Virtual Reality and Assoc. Technologies, in Sharkey, McRindle &Brown (Eds), pp. 19-26, Oxford, UK, 20-22 Sept. 2004.
56. Broeren, J., Georgsson, M., Rydmark, M., Stibrant Sunnerhagen, K., Virtual reality in stroke rehabilitation with the assistance of haptics and telemedicine. Proc. 4th Intl Conf. on Disability, Virtual Reality and Assoc. Technologies, in Sharkey, Sik Lányi & Standen (Eds.) pp. 71-76, Veszprém, Hungary, 18-20 Sept. 2002.
57. Connor, B.B., Wing, A.M., Humphreys, G.W., Bracewell, R.M., Harvey, D.A., Errorless learning using haptic guidance: research in cognitive rehabilitation following stroke. Proc. 4th Intl Conf. on Disability, Virtual Reality and Assoc. Technologies, in Sharkey, Sik Lányi & Standen (Eds.) pp. 77-83, Veszprém, Hungary, 18-20 Sept. 2002.
58. Morris, R.G., Parslow, D.M., Fleminger, S., Brooks, B., Giametro, V., Rose, F.D., Functional magnetic resonance imaging investigation of allocentric spatial memory using virtual reality in patients with anoxic hippocampal damage. Proc. 4th Intl Conf. on Disability, Virtual Reality and Assoc. Technologies, in Sharkey, Sik Lányi & Standen (Eds.) pp. 87-92, Veszprém, Hungary, 18-20 Sept. 2002.
59. Davies, R.C., Löfgren, E., Wallergård, M., Lindén, A., Boschian, K., Minör, U., Sonesson, B., Johansson, G., Three applications of virtual reality for brain injury rehabilitation of daily tasks. Proc. 4th Intl Conf. on Disability, Virtual Reality and Assoc. Technologies, in Sharkey, Sik Lányi & Standen (Eds.) pp. 93-100, Veszprém, Hungary, 18-20 Sept. 2002.
60. Wallergård, M., Cepciansky, M., Lindén, A., Davies, R.C., Boschian, K., Minör. U., Sonesson, B., Johansson., G., Developing virtual vending and automatic service machines for brain injury rehabilitation. Proc. 4th Intl Conf. on Disability, Virtual Reality and Assoc. Technologies, in Sharkey, Sik Lányi & Standen (Eds.) pp. 109-114, Veszprém, Hungary, 18-20 Sept. 2002.
61. Morris, R.G., Kotitsa, M., Bramham, J., Brooks, B., Rose, F.D., Virtual reality investigation of strategy formation, rule breaking and prospective memory in patients with focal prefrontal neurosurgical lesions. Proc. 4th Intl Conf. on Dis-

ability, Virtual Reality and Assoc. Technologies, in Sharkey, Sik Lányi & Standen (Eds.) pp. 101-108, Veszprém, Hungary, 18-20 Sept. 2002.

62. Lo Priore, C., Castelnuovo, G., Liccione, D., Virtual environments in cognitive rehabilitation of executive functions. Proc. 4th Intl Conf. on Disability, Virtual Reality and Assoc. Technologies, in Sharkey, Sik Lányi & Standen (Eds.) pp. 165-172, Veszprém, Hungary, 18-20 Sept. 2002.
63. Maxhall, M., Backman, A., Holmlund, K., Hedman, L., Sondell, B., Bucht. G., Participants Responses to a Stoke Training Simulator. Proc. 5th Intl Conf. on Disability, Virtual Reality and Assoc. Technologies, in Sharkey, McRindle &Brown (Eds), pp. 225-230, Oxford, UK, 20-22 Sept. 2004.
64. Adelola, I.A., Cox, S.L., Rahman, A., Adaptable virtual reality interface for powered wheelchair training of disabled children. Proc. 4th Intl Conf. on Disability, Virtual Reality and Assoc. Technologies, in Sharkey, Sik Lányi & Standen (Eds.) pp. 173-180, Veszprém, Hungary, 18-20 Sept. 2002.
65. Brown, D.J., Shopland, N., Lewis, J., Flexible and virtual travel training environments. Proc. 4th Intl Conf. on Disability, Virtual Reality and Assoc. Technologies, in Sharkey, Sik Lányi & Standen (Eds.) pp. 181-188, Veszprém, Hungary, 18-20 Sept. 2002.
66. Shopland, N., Lewis, J., Brown, D.J., Dattani-Pitt, K., Design and evaluation of a flexible travel training environment for use in a supported employment setting. Proc. 5th Intl Conf. on Disability, Virtual Reality and Assoc. Technologies, in Sharkey, McRindle &Brown (Eds), pp. 69-76, Oxford, UK, 20-22 Sept. 2004.
67. Katz, N., Ring, H., Naveh, Y., Kizony, R., Feintuch, U., Weiss, P.L., Interactive virtual environment training for safe street crossing of right hemisphere stroke patients with unilateral spatial neglect. Proc. 5th Intl Conf. on Disability, Virtual Reality and Assoc. Technologies, in Sharkey, McRindle &Brown (Eds), pp. 51-56, Oxford, UK, 20-22 Sept. 2004.
68. Rose, F.D., Brooks, B.M., Leadbetter, A.G., Preliminary evaluation of a virtual reality-based driving assessment test. Proc. 5th Intl Conf. on Disability, Virtual Reality and Assoc. Technologies, in Sharkey, McRindle &Brown (Eds), pp. 63-68, Oxford, UK, 20-22 Sept. 2004.
69. Leonard, A., Mitchell, P., Parson, S., Finding a place to sit: a preliminary investigation into the effectiveness of virtual environments for social skills training for people with autistic spectrum disorders. Proc. 4th Intl Conf. on Disability, Virtual Reality and Assoc. Technologies, in Sharkey, Sik Lányi & Standen (Eds.) pp. 249-258, Veszprém, Hungary, 18-20 Sept. 2002.
70. Eriksson, Y., Gärdenfors, D., Computer games for children with visual impairments. Proc. 5th Intl Conf. on Disability, Virtual Reality and Assoc. Technologies, in Sharkey, McRindle &Brown (Eds), pp. 79-86, Oxford, UK, 20-22 Sept. 2004.
71. Rand, D., Kizony, R., Weiss, P.L., Virtual reality rehabilitation for all: Vivid GX versus Sony PlayStation II EyeToy. Proc. 5th Intl Conf. on Disability, Virtual Reality and Assoc. Technologies, in Sharkey, McRindle &Brown (Eds), pp. 87-94, Oxford, UK, 20-22 Sept. 2004.

72. Westin, T., Game accessibility case study: Terraformers – a real-time 3D graphic game. Proc. 5th Intl Conf. on Disability, Virtual Reality and Assoc. Technologies, in Sharkey, McRindle &Brown (Eds), pp. 95-100, Oxford, UK, 20-22 Sept. 2004.
73. Lewis-Brooks, A., Interactive painting – an evolving study to facilitate reduced exclusion from classical music concerts for the deaf community. Proc. 5th Intl Conf. on Disability, Virtual Reality and Assoc. Technologies, in Sharkey, McRindle &Brown (Eds), pp. 101-108, Oxford, UK, 20-22 Sept. 2004.
74. Wiederhold, B.K, Wiederhold, M.D., Virtual Reality Therapy for Anxiety Disorders, Advances in evaluation and treatment, American Psychological Association, Washington, 2005. pp. 185-186. and 192-196.
75. Hoffman, H.G., Patterson, D.R., Carrougher, G.J., Use of virtual reality for adjunctive treatment of adult burn pain during physical therapy: A controlled study. Clinical Journal of Pain, 2000;16(3):244-250.
76. Papadogiorgaki, M., Grammalidis, N., Sarris, N., Strintzis, M.G., Synthesis of virtual reality animation from sign language notation using MPEG-4 body animation parameters. Proc. 5th Intl Conf. on Disability, Virtual Reality and Assoc. Technologies, in Sharkey, McRindle &Brown (Eds), pp. 259-266, Oxford, UK, 20-22 Sept. 2004.
77. Takács, B., Kiss, B., The Virtual Human Interface: A Photo-realistic Digital Human, in IEEE Computer Graphics and Applications Special Issue on Perceptual Multimodal Interfaces. September/October 2005
78. Takács, B., Special Education and Rehabilitation: Teaching and Healing with Interactive Graphics, in IEEE Computer Graphics and Applications Special Issue on Computer Graphics in Education. September/October 2005
79. Glassy, D., Romano, J., and Committee on Early Childhood, Adoption, and Dependent Care, Selecting Appropriate Toys for Young Children: The Pediatrician's Role, Pediatrics, 2003; 111(4):911-913.
80. van der Molen, J.H.W., Violence and Suffering in Television News: Toward a Broader Conception of Harmful Television Content for Children, Pediatrics, 2004;113(6):1771-1775
81. Cheng, T.L., Brenner, R.A., Wright, J.L., Sachs, H.C., Moyer, P., Rao, M.R., Children's Violent Television Viewing: Are Parents Monitoring?, Pediatrics, 2004;114(1):94-99.
82. Bandura, A., Ross, D., Ros,s S.A., Transmission of aggression through imitation of aggressive models. J Abnorm Soc Psychol 1961; 63:575-582
83. Bandura, A., Ross, D., Ross, S.A., Imitation of film-mediated aggressive models. J Abnorm Soc Psychol 1963; 66:3-11
84. Bandura, A., Social Learning Theory of Aggression. J Commun 1978; 28:12-29
85. DuRant, R.H., Cadenhead, C., Pendergrast, R.A., Slavens, G., Linder, C.W., Factors associated with the use of violence among urban black adolescents. Am J Public Health 1994; 84:612-617
86. DuRant, R.H., Getts, A., Cadenhead, C., Emans, S.J., Woods, E.R., Exposure to violence and victimization and depression, hopelessness, and purpose in life

among adolescents living in and around public housing. J Dev Behav Pediatr 1995; 16:233-237
87. DuRant, R.H., Treiber, F., Goodman, E., Woods, E.R. Intentions to use violence among young adolescents. Pediatrics 1996; 98(6):1104-1108
88. Flavell, J.H., The development of children's knowledge about the appearance-reality distinction. Am Psychol 1986; 41:418-425
89. Morison, P., Gardner, H., Dragons and dinosaurs: the child's capacity to differentiate fantasy from reality. Child Dev 1978; 49:642-648.
90. Potter, W.J., Perceived reality in television effects research. J Broadcasting Electronic Media 1988; 32:23-41.
91. Wright, J.C., Huston, A.C., Reitz, A.L., Pieymat, S., Young children's perceptions of television reality: determinants and developmental differences. Dev Psychol 1994; 30:229-239.
92. Zimmerman, F.J., Glew, G.M., Christakis, D.A., Katon, W., Early Cognitive Stimulation, Emotional Support, and Television Watching as Predictors of Subsequent Bullying Among Grade-School Children, Arch Pediatr Adolesc Med, 2005;159(4):384 – 388
93. Strasburger, V.C., Donnerstein, E., Children, Adolescents, and the Media: Issues and Solutions, Pediatrics, 1999;103(1): 129-139.
94. Laky, V., Sik-Lányi, C., Using virtual reality in psychology (Virtual worlds in treating agoraphobia and acrophobia), Assistive Technologies – Shaping the Future, G.M. Craddock et al. (Eds.) IOS Press, 2003, pp.628-632.
95. Sik-Lányi, C., Simon, V., Simon, L., Laky, V., Using virtual public transport for treating phobias, Proc. 5th Intl Conf. on Disability, Virtual Reality and Assoc. Technologies, in Sharkey, McRindle &Brown (Eds), pp. 57-62, Oxford, UK, 20-22 Sept. 2004
96. Sik-Lányi, C., Tilinger, Á., Multimedia and Virtual Reality in the Rehabilitation of Autistic Children, Computers Helping People with Special Needs, K. Miesenberger at al. (Eds.) Springer Press, 2004, pp. 22-28.
97. Sik-Lányi, C., Hajnal, Z., Pataky, I., Designing and developing a virtual home for aphasia patients, Assistive Technologies – From Virtuality to Reality, A. Pruski and H. Knops (Eds.) IOS Press, 2005, pp.158-162.
98. Mc Darby, G., Condron, J., Sharry, J., Affective Feedback, Learning skills in the virtual world for use in the real world, Assistive Technologies – Shaping the Future, G.M. Craddock et al. (Eds.) IOS Press, 2003, pp.76-81.

4. Access to Information on Demand by the aid of Digital Talking Books

Thomas Kjellberg Christensen[1] & Margit Dühring[1]

[1] The Danish National Library for the Blind, Teglværksgade 37, DK-2100 Copenhagen, www.dbb.dk, tkc@dbb.dk

Abstract. This chapter addresses the concept and the fundamental ideas of the digital talking book (DTB), with a particular focus on DTBs in the DAISY format. A possible way to structure a digital production and distribution flow is presented, and the way in which this given structure influences the end user's access to information is discussed. In connection to this, the concepts 'Customised end-user product', 'Search and generator machine' and finally 'Server based interactive talking web sites' are described.

1 Equal access to information and the DAISY initiative

Social inclusion is one of the key issues in democratic societies. A basic principle of social inclusion is that all people are to have the same rights and opportunities to participate in cultural, economic and community life. A precondition for the actualisation is to recognise situations in which certain groups are put at a disadvantage and to make a commitment to eliminate inequality and discrimination by facilitating the process of barrier removal to ensure that none are excluded for reasons such as birth, belief and aptitude.

Access to information is a basic human right*, the exercise of which can be severely hampered by the inability to utilise conventional print due to a visual, learning, or neuromotor disability. Traditionally, people with print disabilities – that is, those people who have difficulties reading standard print – have only had access to very inflexible versions of printed material without any real possibilities of reading the text. The limited possibilities of the analogue versions of text material accessible to print-impaired people result in a de facto inequality in access to information.

* The United Nations International Covenant on Civil and Political Rights, Part III, Article 19(2): "Everyone shall have the right to freedom of expression; this right shall include freedom to seek, receive and impart information and ideas of all kinds, regardless of frontiers, either orally, in writing or in print, in the form of art, or through any other media of his choice."

T. Christensen and M. Dühring: *Access to Information on Demand by the aid of Digital Talking Books*, Studies in Computational Intelligence (SCI) **19**, 117–132 (2006)
www.springerlink.com

Dissatisfaction with this state of affairs spurred the formation of the precursor to the DAISY Consortium.

The DAISY Consortium is a non-profit organisation founded in 1996 by a group of talking-book libraries to lead the worldwide transition from analogue to digital talking books. DAISY stands for Digital Accessible Information System.

The vision and mission of the DAISY Consortium are given below along with the organisational membership structure.

1.1 Vision

DAISY's vision is "that all published information is available to people with print disabilities, at the same time and at no greater cost, in an accessible, feature-rich, navigable format" (www.daisy.org).

1.2 Mission

The DAISY Consortium's mission is "to develop the International Standard and implementation strategies for the production, exchange, and use of Digital Talking Books in both developed and developing countries, with special attention to integration with mainstream technology, to ensure access to information for people with print disabilities" (www.daisy.org).

1.3 Organisation

The DAISY Consortium consists of a growing membership of organisations around the world committed to developing equitable access to information for people who have a print disability.

Full and Associate Members of the DAISY Consortium are non-profit organisations, typically national talking-book libraries or national consortia of such libraries. Members of the Consortium actively promote the DAISY standard for digital talking books because it promises to revolutionise the reading experience for people with reading disabilities. Profit organisations are associated as Friends. The DAISY Consortium is managed by a Board consisting of representatives from all Full Member organisations.

The Danish National Library for the Blind is a full member of the DAISY Consortium, and produces digital talking books in the international standard: NISO Z39.86, e.g. DAISY 3.0. The Danish National Library for the Blind has also played an active role in the development of the DAISY standard.

2 What is a Digital Talking Book?

A conventional talking book is an analogue version of a print publication. Traditionally, these audio books are available on cassette tapes, and – in the best of cases – navigation is made possible through low frequency tones that can be heard while winding the tape, e.g. 1 beep might signify a new page, 2 beeps a new paragraph and 3 beeps a new chapter. For very complex texts, such as encyclopaedias, a separate tape is provided with an index for the text and a guide to what the different numbers of beeps signify. This method renders navigation both time-consuming and very demanding on the user, as he or she has to mentally keep track of how many times a certain number of beeps occur before the desired place in the text is reached. Obviously, this solution allows for only the most basic navigation through an analogue text, especially in the case of complex texts. To ameliorate this situation, a forerunner of the DAISY Consortium set out in 1988 to digitise audio books. Today, the DAISY Consortium is continually developing the standard for the particular kind of digital audio books called 'Digital Talking Books'.

2.1 Digital Talking Book building blocks

A Digital Talking Book (DTB, from hereon 'DTB' will denote a digital talking book in the DAISY format) is a multimedia version of a print publication. The rendering of the audio in DTBs can be by human voice, as in the analogue talking books, or in synthetic speech. A DTB can be summarised as a set of digital files that includes:

- one or more audio files containing a human narration of part or all of the source text,
- a mark-up file (explained below) containing some or all of the text,
- a synchronisation file to relate markings in the text file with time points in the audio file; and
- a navigation control file which enables the user to move smoothly between files while synchronisation between text and audio is maintained.

Additionally, the DTB can contain image files. As the standard is to become a multimedia product offering a wide range of features in order to provide services to a broader audience including for example, deaf and hearing-impaired people. A future version will also include video playback capability.

The DTB audio file must be either in WAVE, MPEG-1 or MPEG-2 Layer III (often denoted MP3) or MPEG-4 AAC format.

The text of a book is marked up in XML (Extensible Markup Language), a W3C (World Wide Web Consortium) standard somewhat reminiscent of HTML, the language used for web pages. For use in DTBs the XML mark-up must adhere to a specific DTD (Document Type Definition) defining the 'legal' building blocks of the XML file. The DTD for a DTB is publicly available through the DAISY web pages.

The synchronisation of audio and text is mediated by SMIL (Synchronised Multimedia Integration Language) files, which ensure the correct parallel presentation of the text part and the audio part of a DTB. The SMIL files for DTBs follow a DTD of their own. SMIL is a W3C standard.

The NCC (Navigation Control Center) consists of an NCX (Navigation Control file for XML applications) file, which is an XML application structured in accordance to a separate DTD. The NCX contains navigation points for both text and audio and can be likened to a book's table of contents. Through a SMIL file, each navigation point in the NCX is linked to the corresponding location in the audio and XML textual content files, thus providing direct access to that location. The NCX controls the global navigation and primarily provides access to relatively large parts of the document. The NCX provides an overview of all the points in a text to which a user may navigate and offers direct access to selected structures in the book such as page numbers, notes, figures, etc. Once an NCX item has been selected, local navigation – such as movement within a list or table, or among a group of words, sentences, or paragraphs – becomes possible.

In this way the DAISY DTBs meet the requirements of the talking-book reader by providing access and navigation capabilities to the talking book which have never before been possible to implement in a voice production of a print book. For instance, a blind reader of the DTB can add his or her own notes to the book in the same way a seeing person can write small notes in a printed book. In the DTB the notes are not added by pen or pencil but either in text format or as an oral comment.

2.2 Types of DTBs

DTBs are not required to contain all of the possible constituents mentioned above. The different combinations of elements give rise to the following varieties of DTBs:

- ❖ DTBs containing only linear audio without any accompanying text or any navigation possibilities. The navigation control consists only of the title of the DTB and a link to the start of the audio recording.
- ❖ DTBs containing no audio but instead full structured text and Navigation Center. This kind of DTB can be used for the production of Braille and e-books.
- ❖ DTBs containing full audio and Navigation Center but no text. This kind of DTB has a two-dimensional structure providing both sequential and hierarchical navigation. The structure of these DTBs resembles the table of contents of the print source material. Some of these productions also provide page navigation.
- ❖ DTBs containing full structured text and partial audio. This type of DTB could be used for e.g. dictionaries, where only pronunciations are provided in audio form. The audio components are synchronised with the corre-

sponding text. This kind of DTB can also be used for the production of Braille and e-books.

- ❖ DTBs containing full audio with Navigation Center and partial text. These DTBs have the two-dimensional structure mentioned above. The text components may occur where keyword searching and direct access to the text could be beneficial, e.g. index, glossary, etc. The audio and existing text components are synchronised.
- ❖ DTBs containing full structured audio and text and a Navigation Center. The audio and the text are synchronised. This kind of DTB may also be used to generate Braille and e-books.

The audio parts of the DTBs are rendered with either human or synthetic speech. The types containing text may also include images.

DTBs produced according to the DAISY standard are independent of the distribution medium. The digital master file can be archived and may also be distributed on currently available media such as CDs or DVDs. More importantly, as the technology advances and digital media distribution methods evolve, these same books can be distributed via the newly developed media or system.

2.3 Playing DTBs

There are currently three ways of listening to a DAISY DTB, either through a special DTB hardware player or through special software on a computer or with an MP3 or DVD player. With the MP3 and DVD players it is not possible to use the full structure of the DTB, but the user can listen to the DTB and have a very simple way of linearly jumping forwards and backwards in the book between navigation points. This could be, for example, jumping from paragraph to paragraph, but could also be from a chapter to a page or to a paragraph as these players do not differentiate between the different kinds of navigation points. Additionally, in order to use these two players, the audio files in the DTB should be stored in the right order, which is not always the case. This is not a problem for the special hardware and software DAISY players as the NCC keeps track of the order in which the audio files must be played.

Alternatively, the text part of a DTB can be extracted to yield an e-book. This e-book can be read with assistive equipment such as screen readers and speech synthesis. In this way the user does not necessarily have to invest in a special player to see the titles produced in the DAISY DTB format.

In the DAISY Consortium's work with developing both the standard and the production tools for DTBs, producers of players have been involved from the very start. This means that today there is a range of vendors on the market offering players for accessible material.

Of the various types of DTB players on the market, some are very simple and function very much like ordinary old-fashioned cassette players, and offer a limited choice when navigating the structure of the book. Other players are very sophisticated and enable the user to fully utilise the structure as well as the navigation features of the DTB. For example, to move to a specific page, paragraph, and to insert bookmarks. Some software players display the text on the computer screen in large print, while the text is read aloud. Both software and hardware players are equipped with a default language in which feedback on the player functions in use is given. The content of the DTBs themselves are rendered in the language in which they are recorded.

3 An overview of the digital production flow at The Danish National Library for the Blind

The Danish National Library for the Blind (in Danish: Danmarks Blindebibliotek, DBB) has its roots in the Royal Institute for the Blind, which was inaugurated in Copenhagen in 1811. Since 1924, the DBB has operated as an institution under the Danish State. The agenda of the DBB is to provide equal access to information for print-impaired people.

A front-runner in respect to new technologies, the DBB has not only contributed to the digitisation of audio books but also undergone an internal digitisation process within its own production and distribution.

3.1 Digital production

During the last seven years, the DBB has been deeply engaged in developing concepts and systems for production, storage and distribution of digital products. The vision guiding these activities is that the end user should be able to choose any title in any desired format. It could be an e-book in various formats, on a DTB with audio content or the title could be in the Braille format. An essential idea behind the development of the digital flow has been cost efficiency. Also, it has been of major importance in that upgrading into future formats can be accomplished as smoothly as possible.

The production flow at the DBB beings in a marked up XML source file. Thus, all material produced at the DBB is first marked up according to the part of the DAISY standard that pertains to text. The material is obtained by either scanning the printed text, transforming it from a publisher file or directly downloading it from the Internet. After the mark-up process, the files are stored in an XML database. The end user can then order the material in various formats. The transformation of the source file into the different output formats is done automatically without human involvement.

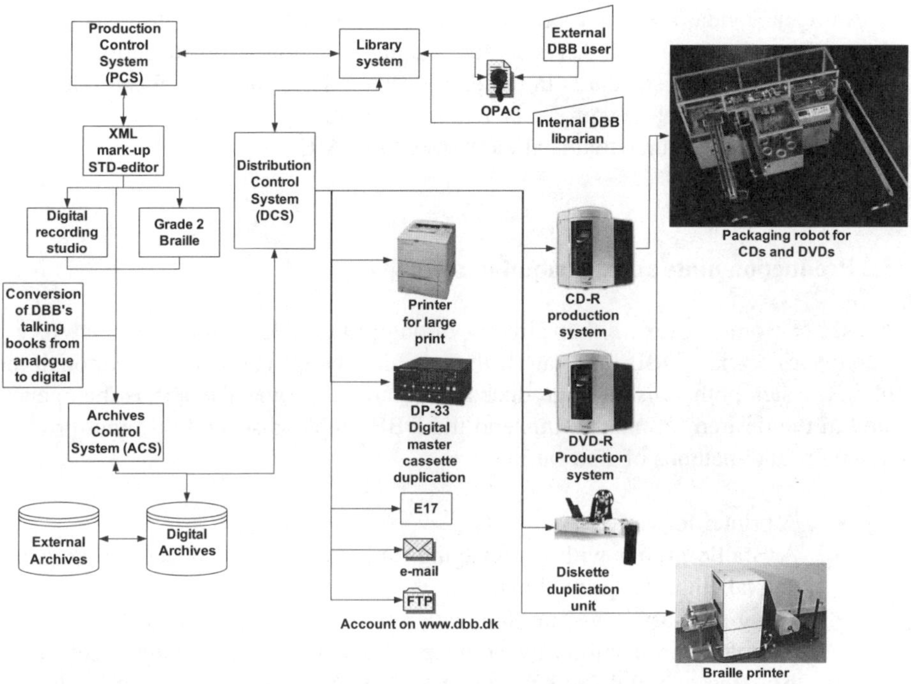

Fig. 1: A schematic overview of the production flow

The formats offered to the end user are the following: Braille grade 0, Braille grade 1, DTBs with synthetic speech and six types of e-books. DTBs with human voice and Braille grade 2 are not part of the automated production flow as both types of material demand a certain amount of human preparation. The production of these two types of material runs simultaneously with the automated 'on demand' service of other formats. The reason why Danish grade 2 Braille cannot be generated automatically is that the rules of contraction for Braille are not logical but are based on semantic rules. Once a Braille book, or a DTB with human speech, has been mastered, it is entered into the digital archive and thereby becomes part of the automated production flow.

The material is stored on servers and is not actually transformed into a readable media until there is a specific demand for a specific book in a specific format. This means that if there is a need to do encryption or to insert a digital watermark or an ID number in the book this can be done specifically for the individual end user. Thus, it is possible to have different forms of encryption or watermarking depending on the kind of material or end-user group served. There may also be different claims from holders of rights for different services or on different types of material.

An open standard for encryption will be incorporated in the DAISY standard in the near future to guard the DTB content against unauthorised distribution. The focus on programming standards in the digital flow allows for the inclusion of external source material for new products, that is, accessible online newspapers and news services where the source text is already stored in XML.

3.2 Production units and distribution methods

A user can order a text, either directly through the OPAC (Online Public Access Catalogue) or via a DBB librarian. If the text already exists it is located through the library system, otherwise it is produced as described above. The text is then generated in the desired format. To this end the DBB employs several different production units and methods of distribution:

- A printer for large print.
- A Braille printer with a packaging unit attached for collecting, wrapping and labelling the printed material.
- A digital master cassette duplication unit for analogue audio books is not part of the production flow at present, but could be readily implemented.
- An internet portal for the direct download of electronic versions by the end user.
- An e-mail distribution system for sending electronic versions to the end user.
- An FTP account system for transfer of the desired files to the end user.
- A CD-R production system that automatically produces ordered materials and labels the CDs with the relevant title and the address of the recipient.
- A DVD-R production system similar to the CD-R production system could be implemented by simply replacing the CD-R drives in the CD-R production system with DVD-R drives should DVD media be preferred.
- A 3/4" diskette duplication unit.
- A packaging robot for CDs and DVDs that automatically handles the entire CD and DVD packaging process is in the planning stages.

Thus, aside from wrapping CDs in envelopes, which is also to be automated in the near future, the process from ordering titles already in the archive to shipping the finished material in the desired format can be fully automated. The modular structure of this production flow allows for easy integration of new production units, distribution methods and future output formats.

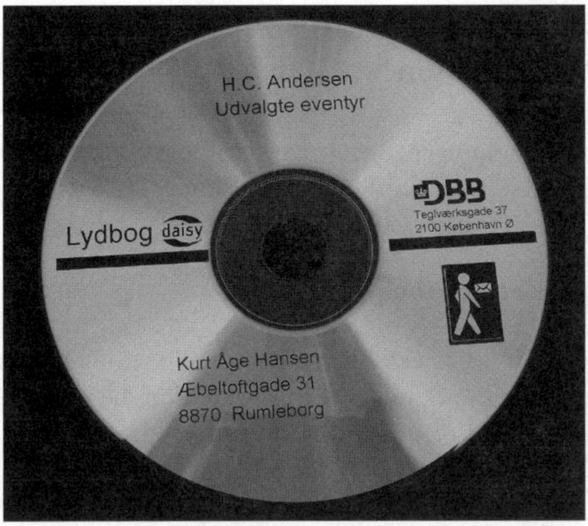

Fig. 2: A DAISY DTB on a CD burned and labelled by the CD-R production system. The label consists of the title of the book and the addresses of both sender and (here a fictional) recipient

With the advent of the 'on demand' digital production and distribution system, the DBB ceased its traditional practice of lending materials, and commenced with a practice where materials are not returned to the DBB, but are instead kept by the user in a 'use and discard' philosophy. One exception is material on cassette tapes, which still follows the circulation of material in a traditional library lending system. The production on cassette tapes will be phased out in the near future and only the 'use and discard' system will remain. This system entails substantial reductions in carriage costs.

The 'use and discard' practice is made possible through the 'Collaboration Agreement' between the DBB on the one side and the Danish Publishers' Association and two Danish writers' associations on the other, with the Danish Ministry of Culture acting as a moderator. The Agreement allows the end users to keep the material provided by the DBB on the condition that the material is rendered illegible and/or inaudible before being discarded. This Agreement is included by reference in the Danish copyright legislation.

The increased efficiency achieved through digitisation and the 'on demand' system also brings about a more cost efficient production flow. Texts are easily accessed, speedily produced and distributed to the end user with a considerable reduction in labour time. The economic resources that are no longer consumed by the production can be used to expand the collection of offered titles.

4 Spin-off products and new possibilities to gain access to information by digitisation

To the advantage of the end user, the structure of a production flow such as the one described above gives rise to several spin-off products.

4.1 Customised end-user product

It is possible for the end user to establish a personal profile at his or her library. This profile describes the layout and presentations in which the end user wants to receive a given type of material and/or title from the library. Below is an example of some of the choices the user will have when defining his or her personal profile. The user may, for instance, choose a certain font and a certain background and text colour scheme. Furthermore, the user can select one or more formats in which he or she prefers to receive the chosen material. In the process of lending out certain material everything is generated on demand. This means that the end user can change the personal profile according to the kind of material he or she wishes to request, and may choose to have magazines in one format and literature in another. It does not cost extra to change between various profiles. The economic resources spent in generating the material are the same regardless of the chosen profile.

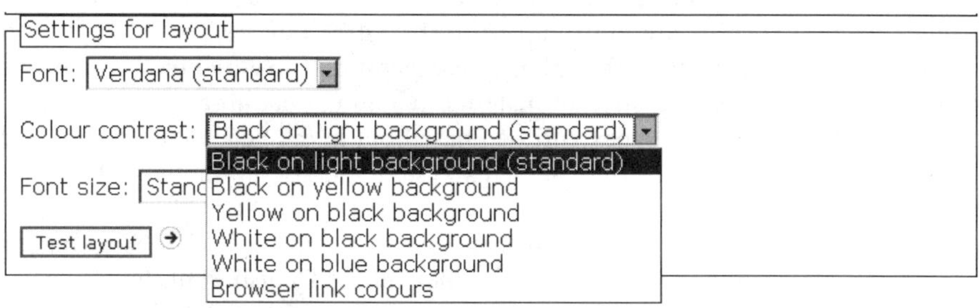

Fig. 3: Layout settings

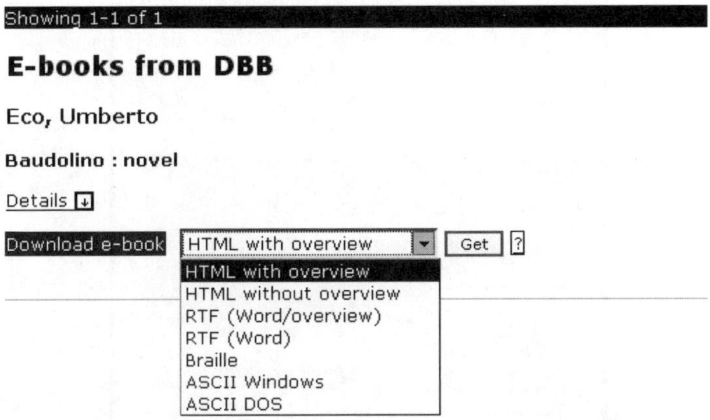

Fig. 4: Formats for e-book download

4.2 Search and generator machine

The ‘Search and generator machine’ service offers the end user the possibility of generating his or her own customised DTB. The user will be able to construct a compendium from the full collection of different titles. The compendium will be based on the texts in which particular search words occur, and the end users can pick and choose which bits and pieces of texts they want to include in a specific compendium. Naturally, the end user will be able to choose a personal format for the compendium.

Below, the various steps in such a search for information about a certain topic are shown. For this demonstration, a search on 'Bill Clinton' is made in the DBB collection. As can be seen, the output of the search shows the various hits that were returned when searching in the DBB collection.

Next step is to decide which of the hits are of interest to a specific compendium, and which structural parts, if not all, of each title should be included in the compendium. Is the whole title or maybe just some selected part, such as chapters or certain sub chapters, of interest?

In this example, one main chapter of the book ‘Terrorisme’, the entire book of the title ’Taletid’ and finally one main chapter from the book ‘Døden fra Lübeck’ are chosen. Once the selection is made and the button ‘Transform’ is clicked, a request is sent to the XML database, and the individual parts of the compendium are selected and transformed into a new compendium. The layout of this compendium will be presented according to the user’s personal profile.

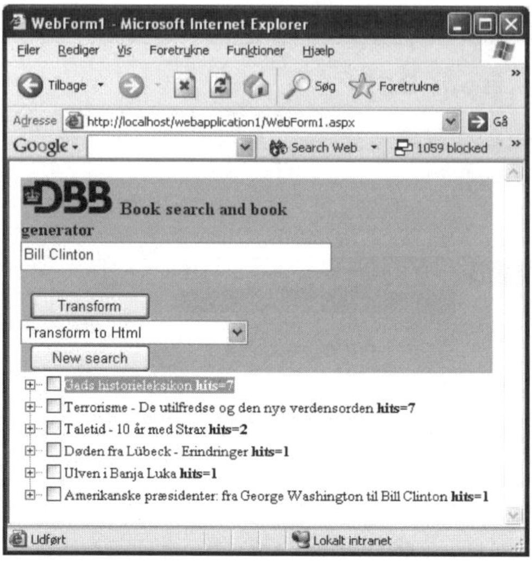

Fig. 5: The search results for 'Bill Clinton' in the collection

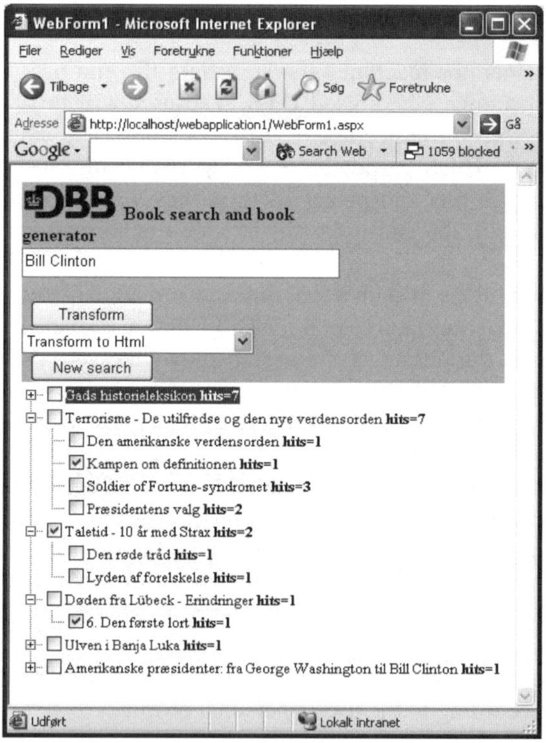

Fig. 6: Selection of parts of the texts from the 'Bill Clinton' search

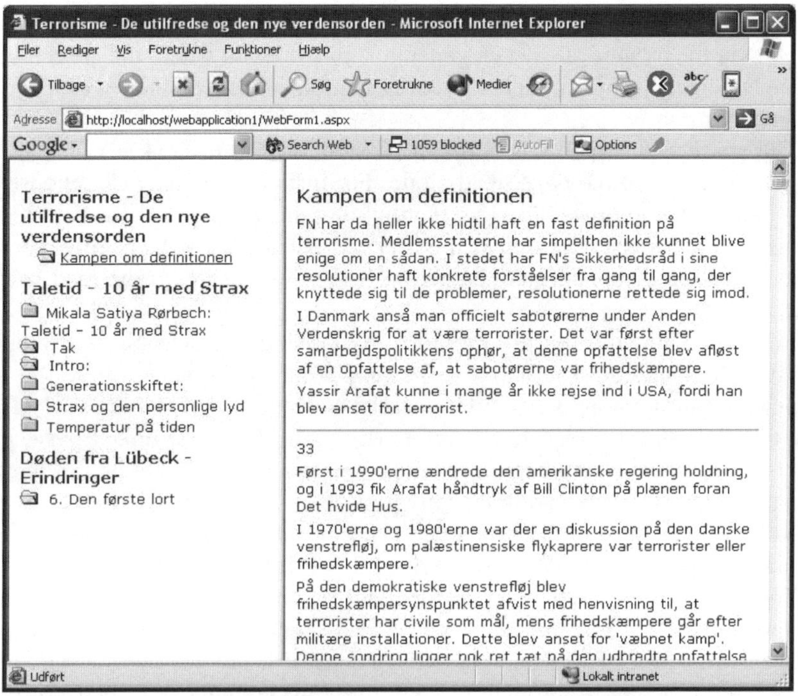

Fig. 7: The new DTB is generated

If the end user wants the compendium as a DTB, it is also possible to generate this on demand with the aid of synthetic speech for parts of the book, which might not have been mastered in human voice.

At present, the 'Search and generator machine' feature exists but is not implemented for public use. This is out of respect for the wishes of the Danish writers' associations. However, such a means of providing structure to collections of texts offers a great potential for assisting users in strong need of highly structured information. Other possible uses of the 'Search and generator machine' could be the embedding of syllabuses in structured systems. That is, those of an entire curriculum at a university could be accessed through this system. It could also be used to access insurance policies in a manageable way, or to provide parts of texts for sale.

4.3 Server based interactive talking web sites and the internet library E17

The 'Server based interactive talking web site' service offers print-impaired people the possibility to interactively navigable web sites by aid of sound. For people who do not have access to screen readers and synthetic speech, the dynamic speech generator developed at the DBB can be utilised to have a web site read out loud. Any computer that is connected to the Internet, runs Internet Explorer and Windows

Media Player and has a sound card and loudspeakers can render online text as speech via the dynamical speech generator. In a domain where the speech generator is implemented, synthetic speech representation of any domain web page can be generated instantly.

The speech generator function can be switched on to have a web page on the domain, or parts of the page, read aloud. For instance, the user can choose to have only part of the text read aloud by highlighting this part, or to have selected words, or maybe only links, read out. If the user has entered some text, for example, on a form, a feature of the speech generator also allows for this to be read back to the user.

Navigation possibilities are provided via tabbing and skip buttons integrated in the speech generator. The text will be read from the point to where the user has navigated. Furthermore, when a link is read out loud it is possible to select and follow this link and the speech generator will continue on the linked page, provided this is also a domain web page. If the link is external, that is, not part of the domain, the speech generator will automatically turn off.

Volume and speed of the synthesised speech can be adjusted to suit the user and, naturally, keyboard shortcuts are provided for all functions.

Technically the speech generator operates on one HTML tag at a time. Only tags containing relevant text are processed. When speech is synthesised for a web page the generator checks whether the text content of a tag has been generated previously. This is achieved through a look up in a list containing a library of all pieces of text for which audio representations have previously been generated. If the speech corresponding to the text been previously generated and stored in an audio file, this file is readily added to a play list. If the text has no audio counterpart, one is dynamically generated using a speech synthesis program and the resulting audio file is added to the play list. In this way an entire web page is matched by a play list containing the audio files in the proper order. This list then plays using the Windows Media Player, thus making the web site talk.

The speech generator is independent of language as this part of the process is implemented entirely through the language of the synthetic speech program, which can be replaced at will.

The dynamic speech generator is implemented on the internet library E17 – "E" which is short for e-books and "17" refers to the section in the Danish copyright legislation that exempts materials for print-impaired people from the normal regulations regarding copyright protection. The similarity to the numbering of European motorways is quite intentional in that the portal is advanced as "the public libraries' motorway to accessible information". The E17 internet library is developed by the DBB in collaboration with the Danish public libraries and several special interest organisations. The E17 portal is a virtual library service through which registered users can search and download accessible materials. Furthermore, E17 is a venue in which the users can interact with one another. That is, recommend books to each other or post messages on the notice board. It is possible for the users to ask a librarian any library-related questions they may have, to use the help pages to navigate the portal and to peruse a guide to other accessible web pages. Integrated in this online library is a number of accessibility features that fulfil the special needs of the specific user group and all web pages can be used with assistive equipment. The E17 internet library includes features not only for blind and partially sighted people, but also for people who are dyslexic, deaf-blind, deaf, hard of hearing, or who have a mental or motor handicap.

The E17 search database not only provides the opportunity to search materials produced by the DBB, but is supplemented by materials registered in the database of the Danish Bibliographic Centre (DBC) containing the Danish National Bibliography of books, journals and other material. Once a week, the titles registered in the DBC database are automatically downloaded to the DBB and filtered in order to select titles of relevance to DBB users. The relevant titles are then included in the E17 database. The material not produced by the DBB can be ordered via a link provided together with the result of the search.

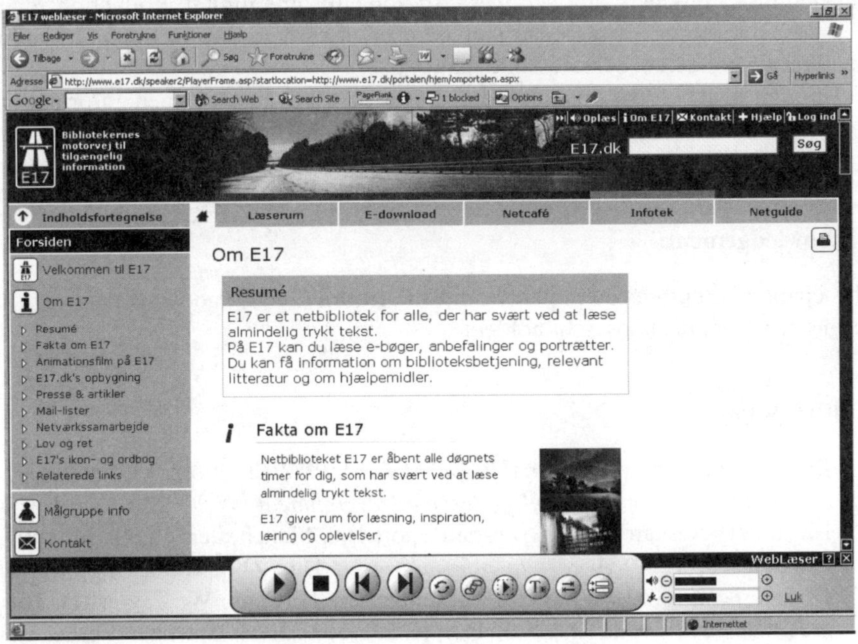

Fig. 8: An E17 web page with open speech generator panel

5 Summary

As described in this chapter, there are some of the significant advantages offered by digitisation to people who have difficulty reading conventional print. This presupposes that the digital potential is recognised and fully utilised.

The development of the international DAISY standard for Digital Talking Books is a prime example of how cutting-edge technology has enabled an enhanced quality of information access for print-impaired people. As an added bonus, the DAISY standard is evolving into a multimedia product, which will be of general interest to the general market.

The implementation of a predominantly automated digital production line at the Danish National Library for the Blind is an example of a functional approach to providing specialised services to a large user group. To the benefit of the users of the library service, the automated digital production line allows for individualised and optimised products and services. Additionally, the digital production reduces pressure on resources, which can then be used elsewhere. For example, to increase the library's collection of accessible material.

Through such efforts, people who are at a disadvantage when information is communicated in standard print are able to make the quantum leap into the digital era in which information can be accessed on a more equal footing than ever before.

Acknowledgement:

This chapter is reproduced in part from Christensen (2004) and www.daisy.org with permission from the copyright holders.

References:

1. Brophy, P., Craven, J.: *Final Report of the REVIEL Project: The Integrated Accessible Library: a Model of Service Development for the 21st Century*. British Library Research & Innovation Report 168. Manchester: CERLIM, 1999.
2. Christensen, T. K.: *Access to Information at Your Own Choice by the Aid of Digital Talking Books*. In: K. Miesenberger, J. Klaus, W. Zagler, D. Burger (eds.): ICCHP 2004, LNCS 3118, pp. 545-551, 2004. Springer-Verlag Berlin Heidelberg.
3. DAISY Consortium (Web Site): http://www.daisy.org
4. Danish Bibliographic Centre (Web Site): http://www.dbc.dk
5. DBB (Web Site): http://www.dbb.dk
6. E17 (the Danish national internet library provided by the DBB): http://www.e17.dk
7. National Information Standards Organisation (NISO) (Web Site): http://www.niso.org
8. World Wide Web Consortium (W3C, Web Site): http://www.w3.org

5 Electronic Locomotion Aids for the Blind: Towards More Assistive Systems

Christophe Jacquet[1,2], Yacine Bellik[2], and Yolaine Bourda[1]

[1] Supélec, Plateau de Moulon, 91192 Gif-sur-Yvette Cedex, France
Christophe.Jacquet@supelec.fr, Yolaine.Bourda@supelec.fr
[2] LIMSI-CNRS, BP 133, 91403 Orsay Cedex, France
Yacine.Bellik@limsi.fr

Abstract. This chapter first presents a review of existing locomotion assistance devices for the blind. These devices are merely proximeters, that measure the distance to the closest obstacles, and convey this information to their users. We introduce the measurement methods (infrared sensors, ultrasonic sensors, laser telemeters) and the user interfaces (sounds and tactile vibrations). Then, we analyse the shortcomings of these systems, and thus explain what additional features new devices could offer. To study the feasibility of such systems, we tackle the different issues raised in the process: localizing users, modeling their environment and adding semantic annotations. Finally, we explain how such devices could fit into a view of ambient intelligence, and how the problems raised extend beyond the field of assistance to blind people.

1 Introduction

According to the World Health Organization, there are 45 million blind people in the world, which amounts to an estimated 1‰ to 2‰ of the population in industrialized countries. This figure cannot be neglected, and the problems encountered by blind people in their everyday life need to be addressed.

In particular, these people are faced with huge difficulties moving in cities, where streets, public transportation systems and shopping malls represent hostile ever-changing environments. As a result, blind people are in danger while moving on their own, and their autonomy is limited.

Indeed, if blind people can generally remember their way to some places, they cannot know in advance what obstacles they will stumble upon. In consequence, the fear of the unknown often leads them to restrict their universe to a small set of known places. They do not dare going anywhere else, thus experiencing limited travel freedom.

Leader dogs can help blind people avoid obstacles and find their way in unknown environments, but they are very expensive: the cost per blind person – leader dog pair ranges from \$15,000 to \$30,000. Despite the financial support of some organizations such as the Lions Club, only very few blind people can actually have a leader dog, while many of them would like to.

C. Jacquet et al.: *Electronic Locomotion Aids for the Blind: Towards More Assistive Systems*, Studies in Computational Intelligence (SCI) **19**, 133–163 (2006)
www.springerlink.com

However, leader dogs represent a very valuable means of dealing with unknown places. Indeed, they see obstacles at a distance, and can therefore anticipate the necessary avoidance maneuvers. In contrast, blind people using canes can feel silent obstacles at a cane's length distance only, so their anticipation capability is very poor [1]. The dog can help them improve their anticipation performances, which leads directly to more fluent trajectories, more self-confidence and easier travel [2].

This is the reason why numerous electronic locomotion assistance systems have been developed. The vast majority of existing systems are obstacle detectors that can warn users of the presence of obstacles *in advance*, so as to enable them to *anticipate* the presence of obstacles and adapt their behavior accordingly. Electronic devices are significantly cheaper than leader dogs, although offering more limited, yet valuable information.

It is important to notice that the white cane is not only a useful obstacle detector for blind people, but also a means by which blind people are recognized by sighted people. In consequence, all locomotion assistance devices for the blind must be designed to be secondary aids, used in complement to the long cane, and not instead of it, because they are not inherently social indicators of blindness.

In this chapter, we first present an overview of existing obstacle detectors, while distinguishing two different facets in these systems: information capture and information presentation. After, we discuss the shortcomings of existing systems and we draw a list of requirements for more advanced systems. Then, we give details about the implementation issues of this new class of systems: user localization and environment modeling, from the structural and semantic points of view. Finally, we show how these issues take place within the broader field if ambient intelligence.

2 Existing techniques

Navigation assistance devices need to deal with two different issues. First, they need to capture contextual information, in general distance information. Indeed, because the basic purpose of these devices is to warn users of approaching obstacles, their basic requirement is to measure distances to obstacles.

Second, they need to present users with this information. The presentation method must be adapted to blind users, and must be suitable for continuous use.

Several electronic travel aids have been proposed that address both of these problems. We have studied the characteristics of a few of them that we think are representative of the available techniques. Below, we present the two problems and the solutions proposed by these devices.

2.1 Information Capture

All current devices only take distance information into account. Thus, they use various kinds of telemeters and proximeters.

Infrared Sensors Infrared sensors are characterized by their quite wide angle magnitude (20 °) which allows the detection of obstacles in the general heading direction of the user. However, their range is limited to a few meters, so they cannot warn users very long before encountering an obstacle.

Tom Pouce (fig. 1), developed by the LAC[3], is an infrared proximeter that can detect obstacles within a 0.5, 1.5 or 3 meters range. Users can select the desired range by means of a three-position switch. Thus they can detect either very close or more remote objects, depending on their current task, for instance following a corridor or trying to find a door in a wall.

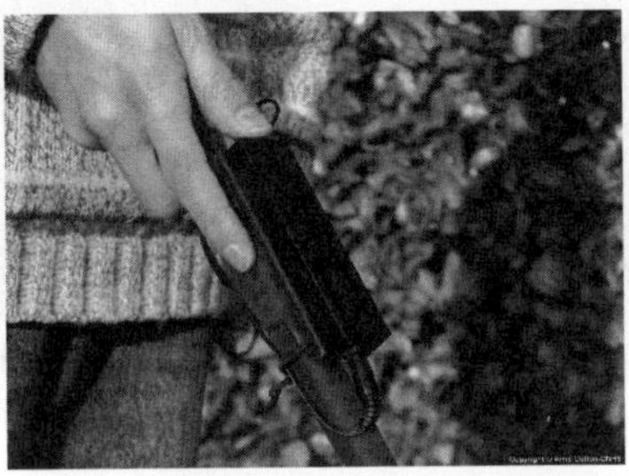

Fig. 1. Photo of the Tom Pouce.

Ultrasonic Sensors Ultrasonic sensors have roughly the same characteristics as the infrared sensors, in terms of range and angle magnitude.

The Miniguide[4], the Polaron[5] and the UltraCane[6] (fig. 2) are examples of mobility aids that use ultrasonic sensors to detect obstacles.

Both devices can be configured to detect obstacles in various distance ranges. The range can be set to 0.5, 1, 2 or 4 meters for the Miniguide, and to 1.2, 2.4 or 4.8 meters for the Polaron.

The Miniguide has got two sensors that should be one above the other while in operation. Thus, users must pay attention to hold their devices vertically.

The Polaron avoids this shortcoming thanks to a neck strap that allows users to wear it around the neck at chest height, thus ensuring a constant ideal position.

[3] Laboratoire Aimé Cotton, Orsay, France.

[4] The Miniguide is a product of the Australian company GDP Research, see `http://www.gdp-research.com.au/`.

[5] The Polaron is a product of the company Nurion-Raycal, see `http://www.nurion.net/`.

[6] The UltraCane, previously known as "Batcane", is a product of the company Sound Foresight, see `http://www.soundforesight.co.uk/`.

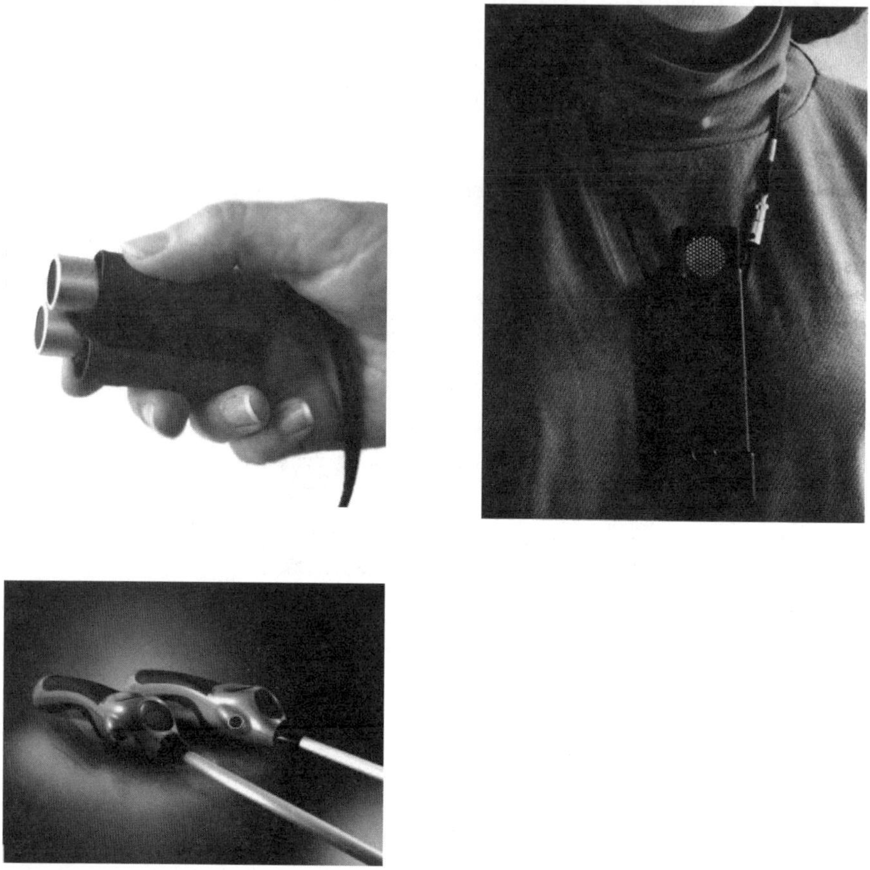

Fig. 2. Photos of the Miniguide (top left), the Ultracane (bottom left) and the Polaron (right).

Laser Telemeters One good example of laser telemeter is the Teletact 1, developed by the LAC.

The distance to the obstacle encountered by the laser beam is measured with about 1% accuracy in the 10 cm – 10 m range. Fig. 3 gives the basic principle of the telemeter [3], and fig. 4 is a photograph of the commercial device. Blind users perceive the direction they point at thanks to the internal awareness of the position of their limbs (proprioception).

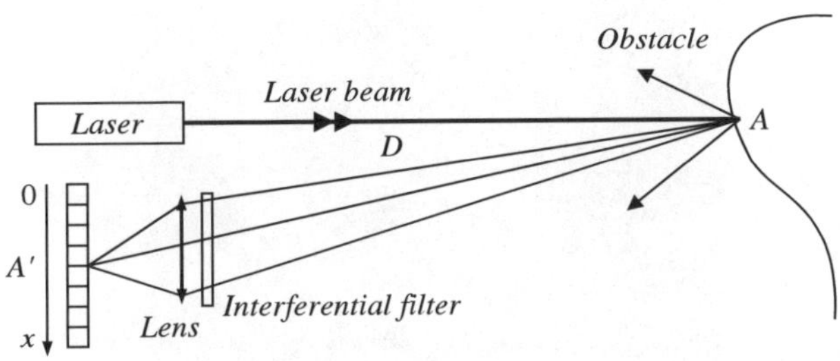

Fig. 3. Basic principle of the Teletact 1's telemeter.

In the device, a laser diode emits a red (670 nm) laser beam that can range up to 30 m (but measurements are precise enough up to 10 m only). For ocular security, the laser power is 1 mW (class II laser product). Thus, there is no risk for passers-by, even if the blind user points the beam at their eyes by mistake.

The beam meets the obstacle at a distance D and creates a laser spot A. The image of the laser spot A through the lens on the CCD line is A'. The position of A' on the line gives the distance D. Actually, $x_{A'}$ is inversely proportional to D, which leads to very simple calculations.

The basic principle is straightforward; the main difficulty is to achieve immunity to diurnal light (up to 200 klux on sunny summer days) that requires the use of some additional optical and electronic systems, such as the interferential filter.

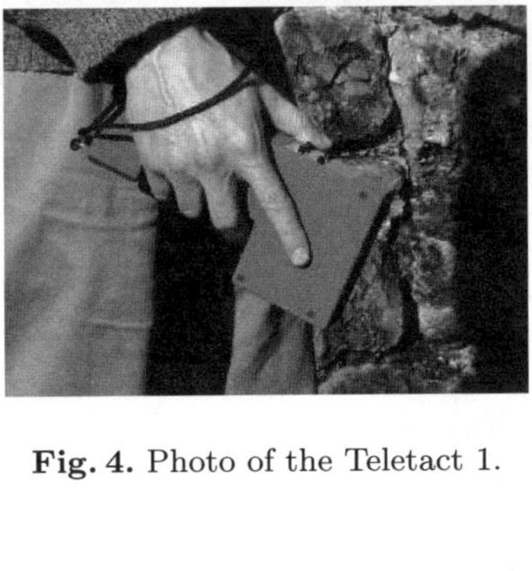

Fig. 4. Photo of the Teletact 1.

The Lasercane N-2000[7] (fig. 5) is quite similar to the Teletact 1. The major difference lies in the fact that the Lasercane is integrated into a traditional white cane, whereas the Teletact 1 is a hand-held device. Thus, the cane can be used as usual, with the electronic aid switched off.

However, the maximum range of the Teletact 1 is greater: 10 m instead of 3.65 m for the Lasercane N-2000.

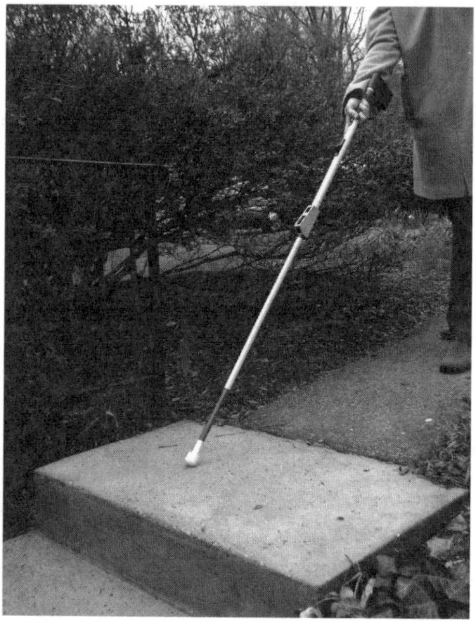

Fig. 5. Photo of the Lasercane N-2000. Photo © by Nurion-Raycal.

Discussion Infrared or ultrasonic devices are more easy to use than laser devices because they have a wide angle magnitude: users just have to point the device in front of them. Conversely, laser devices have a very narrow beam, so users have to scan their environment from side to side, which needs some training and good proprioception capabilities.

There is another issue with laser sensors: their 670 nm laser beam does not generally detect clean windows because it traverses glass without being reflected. Instead, objects located behind windows are detected.

However some users take advantage of this, for example to scan underground stations from train windows. Knowing that windows cannot be detected generally

[7] The Lasercane N-2000 was developed by the company Nurion-Raycal, see `http://www.nurion.net/`.

makes people feel uncomfortable. Black cars with metallic finish pose a similar problem: at high incidences, they do not emit a retro-diffused signal.

However, laser sensors are far more precise than infrared or ultrasonic ones, which gives them an invaluable advantage. That is why the designers of the Teletact 1 have released a new version of their device in collaboration with the LIMSI[8], which, among other things, embeds an infrared proximeter in addition to the original laser telemeter.

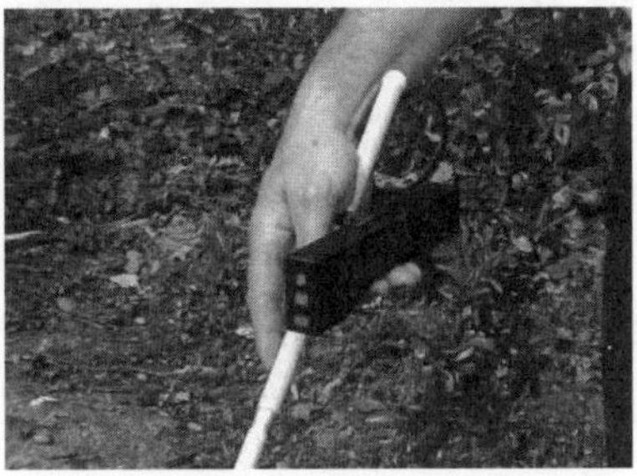

Fig. 6. Photo of the Teletact 2.

The so-called Teletact 2 (fig. 6) is equipped with a strong infrared superluminescent 950 nm proximeter [4, 5]. In case of both proximeter and laser telemetric detection, the system transmits telemeter information. When it senses the proximeter signal only, it sends a "window warning" signal to the user, in order to warn her that she may be approaching a translucent window. The proximeter works within a range of 3 meters, and gives a secured window pane and black car detection up to two meters.

The efficiency of the proximeter is due to the 950 nm wavelength and to the wider angle of the beam (about 20°). Indeed, within a 20° angle at two meters, there is generally some "co-operative obstacle" that can be detected. For instance, when scanning a car, the device detects at least the handles of the doors.

2.2 Information Presentation

Once the distance information has been measured by the device, it must be conveyed to the user in some form. Existing devices use either audio or tactile interfaces.

Audio Interfaces The most simple kind of audio interface is implemented by the Lasercane N-2000: it simply uses a loudspeaker that emits a warning

[8] Laboratoire d'Informatique pour la Mécanique et les Sciences de l'Ingénieur, Orsay, France.

sound when there is an obstacle ahead of the user. As the device also has a tactile interface (see below), audio tones can be disabled in places where sound is restricted (e.g. museums, theaters, etc.)

Thus, the system provides a "go" – "no-go" information about the presence or absence of obstacles. If there is a signal, the traveler should stop. Conversely, in the absence of signal, the traveler may go on.

To convey more detailed distance information, the Teletact 1 uses 28 different musical notes, which correspond to 28 intervals of distance (the higher the tone, the shorter the distance). The 28 intervals of distance are unequal: they are smaller at short distances, because more precision is required for very close obstacles.

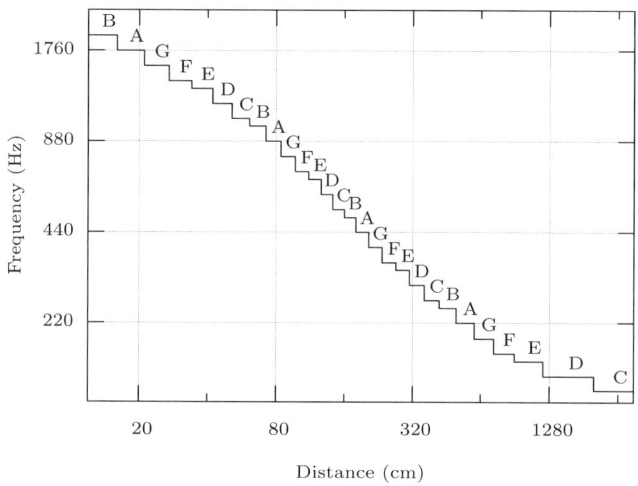

Fig. 7. Correspondence between musical notes and distance intervals (logarithmic scale).

The telemeter itself has a precision of about 1% in distance measurement. Therefore, the number of available musical notes is the limiting factor regarding precision. The device uses flute sounds over four octaves of the major scale (ranging from 131 Hz to 2.1 kHz). So there are 28 useful notes, assigned to 28 unequal intervals of distance in the 10 cm – 30 cm range (see fig. 7).

To get a profile of the obstacles ahead, it is necessary to scan the environment from side to side. It is not important to identify the resulting notes, but to interpret the meaning of the "melody" generated by the environment profile.

Therefore, users must develop some melody interpretation skills beforehand, so as to be able to recognize the melodies associated with common patterns such as corridors, stairs, and so forth. For this purpose, special training sessions have been set up that teach new users how to use their Teletacts.

To avoid confusion between the sounds emitted by the Teletact and possible surrounding noises (for example, coming from a street, or from a crowd), the Teletact uses earphones whose volume level can be adjusted at any moment to keep the distance signal comfortably clear. In addition, this solution presents the advantage of not disturbing the environment.

Some people have difficulties to rapidly merge the audio information with the proprioceptive one (movement of the wrist) to deduce spatial data. This information merge has to become instinctive after learning, because if the person has to think about it, using the device becomes too difficult an intellectual process.

After the necessary training course, fifty blind persons have successfully tested the Teletact 1 and used it to detect obstacles, avoid holes, and to find their way between parallel walls, etc.

The Miniguide has similar characteristics. The audio version uses a tone in earphones to indicate the distance to the closest object: the higher the pitch of the tone, the closer the object. The distance resolution of the audio interface can be set to either 2 cm or 20 cm, which is useful for people who prefer simpler feedback. To find openings only, it is possible to reduce the sensitivity of the system. Finally, there are special *watchdog modes* with very low power consumption used to detect people coming within a 2 meters range.

Tactile Interfaces The audio interface has various defects. Making a difference between musical sounds and street sounds is not a problem, in particular thanks to the earphones and the adjustable audio level. But when the ambient noise level often fluctuates, you have to adjust your proper audio level, and efficient automatic control in this case is very difficult.

To avoid the difficulties inherent to audio interfaces and to shorten the training phase, most devices propose tactile interfaces, generally in addition to an audio interface.

To illustrate this, let us look at the new tactile interface featured by the Teletact 2. It uses vibrating devices located under the user's fingers. Experiments were conducted with two, four and eight vibrating devices, and the four-device solution turned out to be the most successful.

The principle of this method is very simple. Each finger (except the thumb) is in contact with one and only one vibrating device (fig. 8). Each vibrating device corresponds to a distance interval. If an obstacle is detected within one of the four distance intervals, then the corresponding vibrating device is activated.

The Lasercane N-2000's principle is similar, but it stimulates the index finger only.

The Miniguide uses a different approach. In its tactile version, distances are indicated by the speed of vibrations. Thus, distance information is conveyed by the *modulation* of vibrations, not by their *spatial repartition.*

Discussion Using vibrating interfaces seems easier, because perception is more direct and intuitive. That is why beginners generally prefer this. However, people

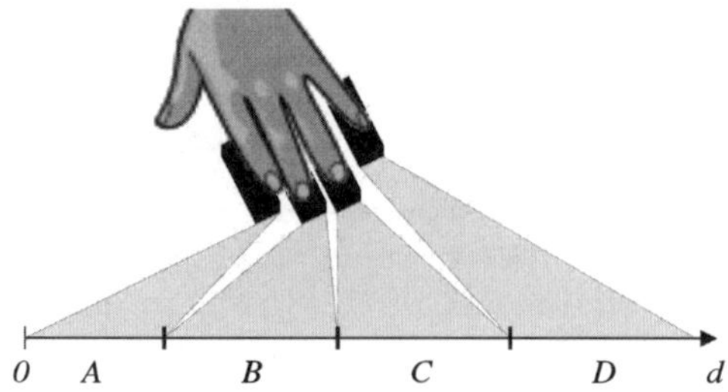

Fig. 8. The four vibrating devices correspond to four distance intervals (*A*, *B*, *C* and *D*).

trained to audio output generally prefer this kind of interface and wish to stick to it because they find it more precise.

As regards the Teletact, the best results to date have been obtained by experienced users with the audio interface. In consequence, the best users tend to choose this solution. But the overall relative performance of the audio and tactile interfaces is not so different, in spite of a number of intervals being reduced from 32 to 4 in the tactile interface.

Furthermore, some advanced users of the tactile interface are beginning to perform tasks previously believed to be possible with the audio interface only (for instance, following a person in a crowd). Ongoing experiments will certainly tell us how these interfaces can be further improved.

However, what seems clear is that both interfaces need a good spatial representation, a good proprioception, and an active attitude: to scan the environment in order to look for obstacles. It is very difficult for blind people from birth to use it because of their lack of spatial representation abilities.

A long training period is required before being able to use a locomotion assistance device in everyday life, and it is especially difficult for elderly people (although there are some exceptions).

The main advantage of theses devices is the good anticipation users obtain and the optimization of navigation. It yields best results with very active blind people who have seen before, with ages ranging from 20 to 40 years old.

Table 1 summarizes the characteristics of the devices presented in this section.

3 Shortcomings of Current Systems

In the first section, we have presented a large variety of locomotion assistance devices for the blind. All these systems share a common characteristic: they only measure the distance to the closest obstacle, and convey it to the user. Their features seem to be somewhat limited when compared to what a leader dog can achieve. The gap is even greater between the mere distance information provided by these systems and the rich information and feedback permanently perceived by sighted people.

Device	Measurement system	Modality	Resolution	Range	Angle magnitude	Autonomy	Learning Time	Size	Weight
Miniguide	ultrasonic	tactile and audio	2 cm	4 m	wide	100 h	not estimated	55 mm × 35 mm × 16 mm	20 g
Polaron	ultrasonic	tactile and audio	binary (absence or presence of obstacles)	1.2 m / 2.4 m / 4.8 m	wide	not known	not estimated	27 mm × 50 mm × 162 mm	257 g
Ultracane	ultrasonic	tactile	not known	a few meters	wide	40 h to 60 h	short time	fits inside a cane	light
Lasercane N-2000	laser	tactile and audio	three levels	3.65 m	very narrow	not known	not estimated	fits inside a cane	450 g (with cane)
Tom Pouce	infrared	tactile	binary (absence or presence of obstacles)	0.5 m / 1.5 m / 3 m	20°	40 h	3 to 4 months (10 to 20 sessions)	55 mm × 75 mm × 17 mm	90 g
Teletact 1	laser	audio	28 levels	10 m	$\ll 1^\circ$	1 h 30 min	6 months (30 hours)	200 mm × 100 mm × 50 mm	450 g
Teletact 2	laser and infrared	tactile and audio	28 levels or 4 levels †	10 m	$\ll 1^\circ$ or 20° ‡	15 h	6 months (30 hours)	170 mm × 50 mm × 20 mm	180 g

Table 1. Summary of the characteristics of existing devices. † 28 levels with the audio interface, or 4 levels with the tactile one; ‡ the angle magnitude is $\ll 1^\circ$ at long range (laser sensor), or 20° at short range (infrared sensor).

This has led us to propose some new features that in our opinion would contribute to making much more usable devices. While these new features would greatly ease the traveling experience of blind people, all current systems lack them.

Thanks to locomotion assistance devices, blind people can avoid running into obstacles. This enables them to gain autonomy in crowded and dynamic places such as streets or train stations. However, people must know the premises beforehand in order to find their way. Indeed, existing devices cannot help people plan their path to some point, nor can they give them information about their location.

For this reason, blind people's autonomy is significantly reduced. When visiting a new place, they must come with a sighted person first, so as to learn how to find their way. Even if when they are sufficiently accustomed to a given place to easily find their way, they often have to ask sighted people to get any additional information. For instance, suppose that Bob is a blind person who regularly walks around an office building. Bob surely knows where the stairs are, so he basically can move alone. However, he surely does not know exactly where Alice's office is located if he has not yet visited her. Since he is blind, he cannot read maps nor signs, so he must resort to asking people at random.

Things can be even worse: if blind people are pushed, they may start to panic and be confused about where they are heading or even where they are located. In this case also they must ask somebody in order to resume walking in the right direction.

Car drivers are faced with the same kind of problem, at a different scale though. Indeed, apart from very well-known directions, it is hard to drive to a given place if one does not know the way. And in the same way as blind people sometimes no longer know their position and direction, car drivers sometimes find themselves driving on an unknown road, to an unknown destination.

As car drivers are concerned, the car industry has come up with a solution. Over the past few years, GPS[9]-enabled car navigation systems have become increasingly popular. They are no longer luxury accessories, but rather quite standard equipment.

A similar solution, adapted to the needs of blind people, would be even more helpful than car navigation systems are for drivers. It would prevent blind people from being completely lost, and guide them to their destination. With a navigation system, blind people could visit new places on their own, with no need of being accompanied by a sighted person.

Even when blind people know exactly where they are, they can be faced with another problem: they cannot easily get information about the surrounding objects. For instance, when in front of a door, they can have no clue as to what is located behind if they do not know beforehand.

In contrast, sighted people can easily get this kind of information: for example, by reading the door sign, they can learn the purpose of the room behind. For instance, an office door generally bears the occupants' names, which is very

[9] Global Positioning System.

important information. The nature of information can even be dynamic: for instance, if an occupant of an office unexpectedly leaves, she can leave a note on the door, stating the reason and the duration of her absence. Or, in the case of translucent doors, a sighted person can know if there is someone in the office simply by noticing whether the lights are on or off.

Since blind people cannot access to this kind of information by themselves, it would be very valuable if an handheld device could give them such pieces of semantic *descriptive* information about places or objects. Where current obstacle detectors can merely tell their users that, says, "there is an obstacle three meters ahead", future devices should be able to add that "this obstacle is a door", and that "this door leads to the boss' office". Advanced systems could be even further precise as to whether the boss is present at the moment or not.

No device of this kind has been released yet. However, now that we have seen the objectives for future assistance systems for the blind, let us summarize the functional requirements for these systems.

A navigation system will need two things:

- a means to know the precise location of the user. There are various localization techniques that will be described in section 4.2,
- structural descriptions of the visited places. For instance, a building will need to be described in terms of rooms, corridors, doors, etc. Section 4.3 will present a framework for environment modeling.

Besides, when giving descriptive information about a place, an information system will have to retrieve *semantic* information associated with it. Section 4.4 will explain how it is possible to store and query semantic annotations.

Structural and semantic descriptions can be either stored on the device itself, or retrieved from an ambient network when needed. We will not detail ambient networks *per se*, since they have become, or at least will rapidly become commonplace. Indeed, different technologies exist, such as third-generation mobile phone networks or ubiquitous WiFi[10] connections inside organization buildings and even at home. We guess that in most places users will very soon have at their disposal *several* different technological solutions to access the network.

4 Requirements for Future Systems

4.1 Introduction: Example of a Next-Generation System

This sub-section introduces a current research project that aims at providing guidance and descriptive information. Although quite limited in regard to the objectives aforementioned, this system is a good starting point for exploring the needs and technological solutions for the design of more complete systems.

[10] Wireless Fidelity. This term informally refers to wireless Ethernet networks, complying with the standards IEEE 802.11a, b and g.

A team of French researchers has launched the RAMPE[11] project [6], which aims at providing an information system for blind people when they take the bus.

Users carry small palmtop devices. For the time being, these devices are simply PDAs[12], on which only three buttons are available to control the system. This prevents blind users from confusing among many different buttons.

While walking in the streets, when a user comes close to a bus stop, his PDA pronounces the name of the bus stop through speech synthesis. If the user is interested in the given bus stop, she pushes a button. Then, the PDA requests the bus stop to advertise its position: a loudspeaker situated atop the bus stop emits a sound that the user is normally able to locate.

When the user arrives at the boarding location, his PDA reads the names of the corresponding lines. If the user shows her interest for a given line, the PDA reads the name of the stops on this line.

Technically speaking, the system is based upon WiFi access points[13] located in the bus stops. The *context of use* of the handheld device is simply the set of bus stops nearby. The detection of the latter is straightforward: the system just has to get the list of accessible WiFi access points, which is done by performing a standard WiFi scan. Therefore, when the user selects a bus stop, it is tantamount to selecting a WiFi access point. The device only needs to connect to it and use the resulting network connection to retrieve information (e.g. the line maps) or send commands to the bus stop (e.g. the command to advertise its position through the loudspeakers).

This system is currently being tested in urban bus lines. It is likely to be highly beneficial for blind people, because they can move around the lines and take buses without having to rely on passers-by. Indeed, they can know where to wait for a bus, which bus to take, and when to get off. This will improve their autonomy.

However, this system cannot be used in any place, as it relies on a very specific infrastructure installed in the bus stops. Indeed, the system does not just use any available WiFi network: it requires the access points to be installed in the bus stops, because WiFi access points coverage is used as a bus stop proximity sensor. Thus this system, although very well suited for its purpose, cannot easily be transformed into a *general* purpose guide for blind people.

A general purpose guide might as well rely on the presence of a wireless network, because such networks are becoming commonplace. However, one such guide cannot reasonably require *constraints* on the top *topology* of the wireless network.

---

[11] Référentiel d'assistance aux personnes Aveugles pour leur Mobilité dans les transports publics et des Pôles d'Échanges, see `http://www.esiee.fr/~rampe/`

[12] Personal Digital Assistant.

[13] A wireless network is built around so-called *access points* that route data packets and act as beacons for network discovery and identification. Each access point has a unique identifier.

In this section, we introduce the requirements of future systems, in terms of user localization, environmental and semantic modeling. We introduce the concepts from a general point of view, although we will sometimes give more detailed information because we have already worked on implementing such a system.

4.2 User Localization

Introduction Several techniques have been proposed to track user location. To compare them, [7] proposes several discriminating criteria :

- *geographic vs symbolic*: some systems perform *geographic positioning*: they provide geographic coordinates with respect to a given coordinate system. Conversely, other systems perform *symbolic positioning* : they provide references (e.g. identifiers) to known objects. For instance, if Alice is in her office, a positioning system would yield the coordinates "`45° 34' 26'' N, 1° 47' 52'' E`" in the former case, and the identifier "`alices_office`" in the latter case,
- *absolute vs relative*: when performing *absolute positioning*, positions are given with respect to a fixed coordinate system. Conversely, when performing *relative positioning*, positions of points are given with respect to each other,
- *locality*: calculations can be performed locally, on a device carried by the user (*local localization*), or at the level of the surrounding infrastructure (*global localization*). In the former case, each positioning device keeps track of its own current position, whereas in the latter case, the infrastructure keeps track of the position of all users,
- *accuracy* measures the typical error of the system. For instance, a given system can have an accuracy of 10 meters, which means that *most of the time*, the position it reports is within 10 meters of the real position
- *precision* quantifies how often the positions reported by a positioning system are within the system's accuracy. For instance, if the former system has a precision of 95 %, it means that reported positions are within 10 meters of the real positions *95 % of the time*,
- systems can be designed to operate at different *scales* : worldwide, countrywide, inside a given building, etc.,
- system *costs* greatly vary. System designers must reach a trade-off between cost and precision and accuracy requirements.

Let us now examine the main positioning techniques that have been proposed (triangulation, proximity sensing, scene analysis, dead reckoning), and their technological variations. In a later sub-section, we will see how it is possible to increase precision and accuracy by combining *several* of these techniques.

Triangulation To perform triangulation, a system must know the positions of known reference points. It can then either measure the distances to these points (the technique is then called *lateration*), or the angles to these points (the technique is then called *angulation*). Such systems try to calculate coordinates : they are *geographic positioning* tools. Diverse techniques can be used to obtain the measurements.

The most common way is to install a radio-frequency beacon on each reference point. This way, users carry a positioning device (*local localization*) which measures distances by estimating the transmission time of travel, or by measuring the attenuation of the signal, which can then be used to deduce the position of the positioning device.

GPS is a well-known system that relies on triangulation. The reference points are satellites which move. The user receiver knows precisely the satellite trajectories, hence their position at any time. Satellites are precisely synchronized with each other and carry atomic clocks. The messages they send are time-stamped. User receivers measure *pseudo-distances*. That is the difference of the time-of-flight between the signals received from the satellites. This way, receiving the signals from three satellites suffices to calculate the two-dimensional absolute position. For three-dimensional positioning, a fourth satellite is needed.

GPS offers an accuracy of a few meters, especially since "Selective Availability[14]" has been turned off. However, GPS will work reliably only if at least four satellites are visible and have strong signals. This poses no problem in the open, hence the success of GPS among hikers and car drivers. Unfortunately, when users in cities are surrounded by high buildings the reception of satellite signals tends to be difficult. This phenomenon, called the *canyon effect* [8], often prevents reliable positioning by GPS in cities.

Inside buildings, the situation is even worse, and generally, GPS signals are very weak, and thus not usable. It is nevertheless possible to install a "constellation" of pseudo-GPS satellites (actually, beacons) inside a building. If the characteristics of pseudo-satellites are identical to these of actual GPS satellites, it is possible to use standard GPS receivers inside the building. This solution may be costly, because GPS signals are quite difficult to generate. Other solutions may be adopted, and are based on slightly modified GPS receivers [9].

It is also possible to use the same kind of triangulation techniques as used by GPS, but using other kinds of timestamped beacons, such as mobile phone base stations.

Triangulation-based location systems for mobile phones will be implemented shortly in the US, because the FCC[15] has passed rules for an Enhanced-911 service (E-911 Phase II) that will oblige telephone networks to be able to locate mobile phones within 50 to 300 meters when users call 911. Different techniques will be used. These include GPS (local localization), measurement of the angle of arrival (AOA) or time difference of arrival (TDOA) of mobile network beacons (local localization), and enhanced observed time difference (E-ODT). The latter

[14] Selective Availability was a "feature" of the GPS system that prevented people not accredited by the US Department of Defense from accessing the system's full accuracy. In practice, civilian users could only access deteriorated signals.

[15] Federal Communications Commission.

system requires additional beacons to be installed in mobile networks, but the positioning is ultimately performed locally by handsets.

Other systems are based on signal strength measurements in wireless networks, for instance mobile phone networks or WiFi networks. These systems can perform either local or global localization. This is because both fixed points (mobile phone base stations and WiFi access points) and mobile units all transmit signals. For instance, Microsoft's RADAR system achieves local localization by measuring the signal strength and signal-to-noise ratio of WiFi signals. However, these techniques remain imprecise due to uncertainties in radio propagation models [10] and signal strength measures.

All the solutions evoked earlier achieve absolute positioning. However, recent research work has been done in the field of UWB[16] communications [11]. In these systems, a vast quantity of users carry so-called UWB transceivers that communicate with each other and measure distances to one another. By exchanging their measures, the whole set of UWB transceivers can calculate their respective positions (*relative positioning* performed *at a global level*, due to algorithms distributed across the network of UWB transceivers).

Proximity Sensing The first commercial system of this kind was introduced by Olivetti in the early 1990s. It was called *ActiveBadge*. People had to wear badges that emitted their unique identifier through infrared signals every ten seconds. Infrared receptors were installed in each room, and constantly waited for badges to send their identity. This positioning system is symbolic and global. Location is done by room identifiers and is performed by the infrastructure.

A similar system has been introduced with Bill Schilit's ParcTab system [12, 13]: people carry PDAs that use an infrared-based computer network built around beacons installed in each room. By keeping track of the beacon currently in use to communicate with a given ParcTab device, the infrastructure can track the location of users.

In the CyberGuide system [14], infrared beacons are installed in rooms, and mobile devices perform local localization by identifying the nearest beacon.

Ultrasonic signals can be used in a similar way as infrared signals. For instance, the *ActiveBat* system, developed by AT&T (formerly Olivetti Research) in 1998, relies on ultrasound badges worn by people. Grids of ultrasound receivers are installed in the ceilings of rooms, thus providing a geographic location service by measuring the transmission time of ultrasonic signals. Conversely, in the *Cricket* system receivers are worn by users, and rooms are fitted with arrays of ultrasonic beacons. The main impediment to the massive adoption of these systems is their cost as many devices have to be installed in the environment for them to work.

Radio networks can also be used to sense the proximity of stations, although they do not try to perform triangulation as in the former sub-section. For instance, E-911 Phase I only uses the base station identifier as handset location.

[16] Ultra Wide Band.

Users are symbolically localized to a given cell of the mobile phone network. Similarly, a WiFi-enabled device can be localized by giving its access point identifier (ESSID, Extended Service Set Identification). Likewise, Bluetooth devices can "feel" the presence of each other by just scanning the Bluetooth devices located nearby.

RFID[17] is a technology that enables the detection of most generally passive tags. An antenna sends radio-frequency waves to the tags, which provides enough energy for them to answer by giving their unique identifier. This technology is used in such applications as identifying people when they enter buildings, tracking parcels when being routed for example [15].

Therefore, if an area is equipped with an RFID reader, it can detect people passing by, provided that (a) everybody wears an RFID tag, and (b) that the reader is sensitive enough. In this case, people positioning is mandatorily carried out by the infrastructure. Tags have to be installed in every "semantically-significant" place [16], and a server can then keep track of all users.

Conversely, it is possible to install tags at key locations in the environment and to equip user devices with tag readers. In this case, localization is performed at a local level. There is no need for the infrastructure to be computer-enabled; disseminating passive tags is sufficient. When passing by an RFID tag, a user is notified that she enters the corresponding area.

In these two examples, RFID tags are used to perform *symbolic* localization. A tag or a tag reader is in every place of interest, which allows identification. Studies have shown that it is possible to perform *geographic* localization as well by measuring the strength of signals received from the RFID tags [17].

Some issues arise with RFID technology, such as interferences between tags or between tags and metallic objects [18]. However, these problems can be overcome [19], so that RFID provides a reliable way of identifying objects by proximity sensing.

We have seen in subsection 4.2 that the strength of WiFi signals, with a propagation model, could be used to perform triangulation. However, as we have seen, this technique is unreliable. It is possible to use WiFi signal strength to perform localization without resorting to triangulation. At every point of a building, one can measure and record the strengths of the signals received from access points in a database. This way, a "fingerprint" is associated with each point. When someone wishes to know his position, he can measure the fingerprint of his present location, and look up in the database to find the closest recorded fingerprint, which gives the location.

This technique enables *geographic localization* through WiFi proximity sensing. This is not just symbolic localization with respect to the nearest access point. Commercial products of this kind have been developed by companies such as Skyhook Wireless[18] and Ekahau[19]. Intel's Placelab[20] uses a similar system, but

[17] Radio-Frequency Identification.

[18] `http://www.skyhookwireless.com/`.

[19] `http://www.ekahau.com`.

[20] `http://www.placelab.org/`.

it is applied to both WiFi access points, cellular phone beacons and Bluetooth devices, and not just to WiFi cells [20].

It is even possible to use FM radio stations as beacons, and this was demonstrated in Microsoft Research's RightSPOT system [21]. This system measures and ranks the signal strengths of several commercial FM radios. A database holds the probabilities of the possible rankings for each location. For a given ranking, a Bayesian classifier provides the most probable location. This system has limited accuracy: it can only precisely determine the suburb.

Scene Analysis These systems are based on video cameras and computer vision software. Cameras constantly take pictures of the rooms, and the processing power located in the infrastructure tries to identify people. A good example of theses systems is Microsoft Research's *Easy Living.*

People identification can be performed thanks to facial recognition. For instance it is possible to combine several modalities such as silhouette, skin color or face pattern. However, ambiguities can more easily be eliminated if people or objects have attached labels specially suited for computer vision, such as two-dimensional bar codes.

Dead Reckoning and Map Matching When no infrastructure such as GPS is available for position tracking, a device can independently try to keep track of its own position unaided. The basic idea is to embed an inertial unit that constantly measures the acceleration vector of the device, and then try to compute the device's position by integrating the acceleration twice. This method is called *dead reckoning.* Using this method, new positions are determined in a *relative* fashion, by estimating how far the user has moved since the last known absolute position. For example the last known position could be obtained from the GPS before it lost the signal.

Unfortunately, dead reckoning is very error-prone [22]. Computed positions are likely to deviate from the real positions because of cumulative errors due to the two successive integrations of the signals. To overcome this shortcoming, the *map-matching* method [23] suggests that the movements of people are restricted along well-defined paths on a map. Hence, it is possible to reduce deviation errors by computing the most probable position of the user *along a path* and not in every possible direction.

Map matching is used in car navigation systems, both in those relying on GPS as well as those relying on dead reckoning. This works well for car drivers because they are forced to follow roads, but in case of pedestrians movements are less predictable, especially in open spaces outside buildings.

Map matching is also extensively used in the field of robotics: even in robots that do not embed an inertial unit, the system precisely knows which actions the robot has made. Every moving and stirring command applied to the motors is kept in memory. Hence, the trajectory can be re-constructed and corrected by matching it against a map.

However, these techniques do not apply so well to human beings because of a number of factors.

1. when walking, human beings tend to not necessarily follow paths or roads, but rather walk around them. Especially in the case of blind people, users sometimes walk away from a "normal" path. As these are precisely the cases when assistance devices will be the most useful, they *must* keep track of people even when they adopt "abnormal" behaviors,
2. the human body is not as solid as a robot or car chassis. In consequence, if an inertial unit is attached to a human being, it will be tilted in every possible direction, its height will vary, and so on. All this is prone to large errors accumulating.

Combination of Several Techniques Each of the techniques presented in these sections has its own advantages and disadvantages. However, when several positioning techniques are available simultaneously, it is possible to increase the global accuracy and precision by combining their results.

For instance, if several geographic positioning techniques are simultaneously available, such as GPS data and WiFi triangulation the information can be fused. This can be done either by averaging them, or by using more advanced techniques such as Kalman filters.

Likewise, geographic localization and symbolic localization can be used in a complimentary manner. This way, it is possible to track the position of objects through computer vision (geographic localization), and to give a label to these objects when detecting their RFID tags or to a WiFi access point that they may carry [10].

4.3 Environment Modeling

To be able to locate users within their physical environment, a system must have a model of that environment. So far, we have worked on building descriptions only. However, the concepts introduced here can be extended to cover the full range of environment descriptions. This section explains how it is possible to represent the structure of buildings in a way that makes sense to a context-aware assistance device for the blind.

Existing Solutions Current formats for 3D scene description (such as VRML [24] or X3D [25]) focus on describing the mere visual *appearance* of environments. Indeed, they target *sighted people* and try to render scenes with as many visual details as possible. In contrast, we target *blind people* and thus we need to model the *structure* and *semantics* of environments.

The *structure* of architectural environments determines how architectural elements are organized to compose buildings. Structure is either visible (e.g. walls) or invisible (e.g. frontiers dividing a room in several zones, for instance smoking ones and non-smoking ones). These invisible frontiers are at least as important as the visible architectural elements. Therefore, they *must* be represented in the model, which 3D scene description formats do *not* take into account.

For data storage, geographical databases [26] represent an interesting framework. However, they do not allow *explicit* representation of structure, so we will not use them for building description.

Modeling Building Structure We have devised our own means to describe the structure of buildings. It allows descriptions to be built in a hierarchical fashion. Later we will see that such descriptions can be represented as XML[21] data. Our model is three-tier:

- *first tier:* we call *lexical elements* the simple (elementary) architectural elements, such as walls, doors, flights of stairs, and so on. Lexical elements are not necessarily *physical* elements. For instance, to delimit two zones in a room (say, a smoking one and a non-smoking one), we may define a *"virtual wall"* that is just like a wall, except that it has no physical existence;
- *second tier:* so-called *syntactic elements* are complex architectural elements, formed of several lexical elements. For instance, a room is defined by its walls, a stairway is defined by several flights of stairs and landings;
- *third tier:* syntactic elements are further aggregated in what we call *aggregation elements.* For instance, several offices can be gathered in a *cluster* called, say, "sales department".

A given description is composed of various elements that are instances of more general concepts. For instance, the laboratory's door is an instance of the general concept of a door. These concepts (or classes) take place in a concept hierarchy whose main branches correspond to the three families of objects.

All classes derive from an abstract common ancestor called an `Element`. This class has got three abstract subclasses, corresponding to the three tiers of our model: respectively `Lexical Element`, `Syntactic Element` and `Aggregation Element`. Concrete classes are then derived from one of these abstract classes, depending on what tier they belong to.

In a description, objects from the three tiers are bound together by two kinds of edges (cf. figure 9):

- *inclusion links* (solid lines) represent geometric inclusion between elements within a given tier;
- *composition links* (dotted lines) enable objects of tier n to be composed of elements of tier $n-1$.

For instance, on figure 9, office number 2 is included in floor number 1. In turn, the later could be included in a given building.

As for composition, office number 2 is said to be composed by several walls (`w_1`, `w_2`, etc.). In other words, these walls *define* and *geometrically delimit* the office.

[21] eXtensible Markup Language.

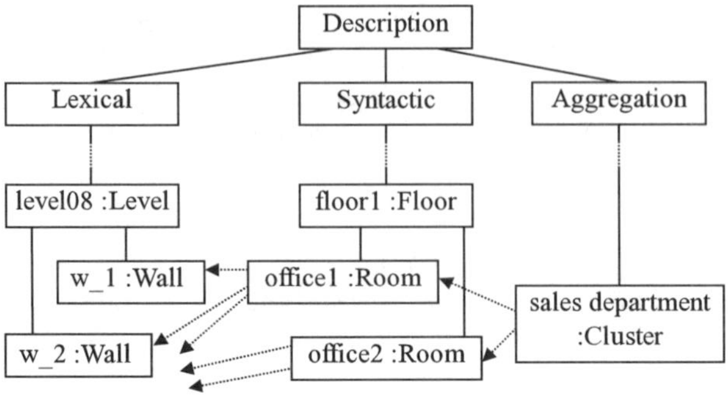

Fig. 9. Excerpt of an example description. The *sales department* is composed of two offices, which is in turn defined by some walls, and is included in a floor.

Representation of Descriptions This model has a strong hierarchical structure, so it is natural to use a representation format that makes this structure explicit. XML allows this type of explicit representation of structure, in addition to being widespread and universal. Therefore, we can use XML to store the three tiers of a description. For instance, the description of fig. 9 would lead to the following XML file:

```
<Description>
  <Lexical>
    ...
      <Level id="level-08" z="16m" height="2.20m">
        <Wall id="w-1" x1="2.3m" y1="4.2m" ... />
        <Wall id="w-2" x1="2.3m" y1="4.2m" ... />
        ...
        <Wall id="w-n" x1="12.3m" y1="13.2m" ... >
          <Door id="d-1" x="2.3m" width="1m" ... />
          <Window id="f-3" x="2.7m" y="0.5m" ... />
        </Wall>
      </Level>
    ...
  </Lexical>

  <Syntactic>
    ...
      <Floor id="floor-1">
        <Room id="office-1">
          <link ref="w-1" />
          <link ref="w-2" />
          ...
        </Room>
        <Room id="office-2" />
```

```
          ...
          <link ref="w-n" />
        </Room>
      ...
  </Syntactic>

  <Aggregation>
    ...
      <Cluster id="sales-department">
        <link ref="office-1" />
        <link ref="office-2" />
      </Cluster>
    ...
  </Aggregation>
</Description>
```

Inclusion links are represented implicitly through XML element imbrication, while composition links are represented explicitly thanks to XML `link` elements.

Relevant Information Using architectural descriptions like these, a locomotion assistance device will be able to determine where the user is. Then it will be able to provide the user with information located at the corresponding node.

However, we wish to give users the possibility to designate an object with a pointer, so that the system provides relevant information about the *pointed object* and not about the user's current location or nearest object.

Technically speaking, determining the pointed object is relatively easy if one already knows the *geographic* coordinates of the user. We can use a laser telemeter as a pointer. This way, with a compass and an inclinometer, one can calculate the trajectory of the laser beam, and thanks to telemeter data, one can finally deduce where the point of interest is.

Then, the whole issue boils down to determining the *level of detail*, i.e. the *granularity* of information needed by the user about the pointed object.

Indeed, too general information is useless, and too detailed information might not be understandable if the user does not know the associated context. To illustrate this, let us look at an example (see figure 10).

Suppose that a user is located on the second floor of the Computer Science (CS) Laboratory. She points through the window at an office on the first floor of another building, the Library building, located next to the CS building. What information shall we return? Information attached to the room, the floor, the building, the campus...?

If we provide the user with information about the campus, it will be far too general, and thus prove totally irrelevant, hence disturbing for her. Conversely, if we give her details about the very office at which she points at, (a) she will lack the context to understand this information, and (b) she surely is not interested

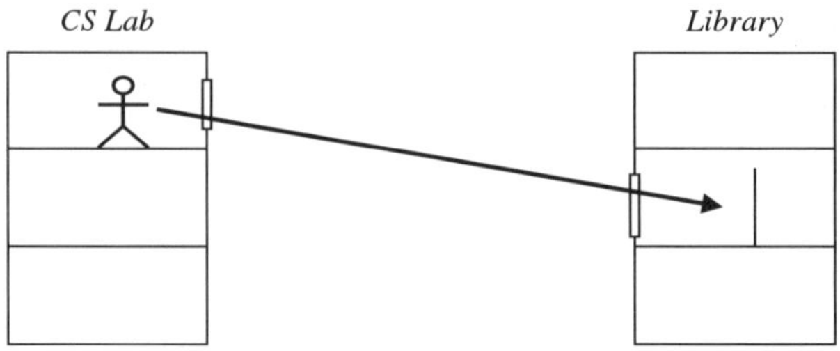

Fig. 10. A user points from one building to another one.

in an *office* located in another building anyway. In consequence, we must provide her with an intermediary level of information.

To solve this problem, we have devised an algorithm to determine a relevant level of information granularity.

We represent the scene as a tree (see figure 11): the user is located in u, and the pointed object in p. First, let us find the deepest node that is common to both the path leading from u to the root, and the path leading from p to the root. This node is labeled c on Fig. 11.

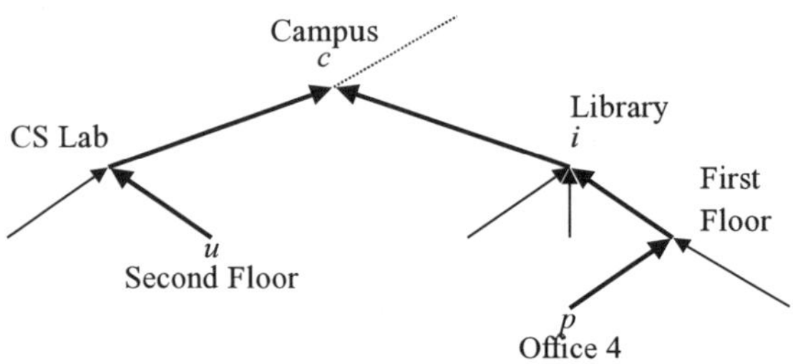

Fig. 11. A tree formally describing the situation depicted on figure 10.

What happens if we return information located at c or above? Such information is too general, because it covers p as well as u. Thus, it will probably be useless for the user, because being in the CS building they already know that they are on the campus.

In consequence, we should return information located *below* c. Therefore, this information will be on the sub-path leading from p to c since it must describe p. But it must be within the context of the user, because they could not understand it otherwise.

Therefore, we return information located in i, i.e. the most general information on the sub-path leading from p to c. This corresponds to a *default granularity level*.

A locomotion assistance device may use this algorithm to determine the level of information granularity provided as a default in the interface. However, the user may wish to retrieve information located at another level. For this reason, the final user interface will offer some means of climbing up and down the tree, thus providing her with either more or less details about her object of interest.

4.4 Beyond Structure: Semantics

Motivation With the techniques described so far, one can design a handheld device that keeps track of the position of the user, and thus is able to locate her on a structural description of the environment. Moreover, when the user points in a given direction, we are able to determine a default object which is likely to correspond to a level of information granularity that makes sense to her.

The objects manipulated by the system (whether corresponding to the location of the user or to a designated direction) are structural elements (for instance, doors, rooms, etc.) A system can know these elements and their characteristics, and thus provide relevant information to the user: for example, "this is a door; and you have to push it to go beyond". For another door, the system may know that the user has to pull it open.

However, the user may be interested in getting additional *semantic* information. In the above example, the system would not only state that the user is standing before a door: it would add that this door leads to an office, and would then give out the office owner's name, the office function, and so on.

To do this, one may wish to associate semantic information to the structure description. More generally, such information can be used:

- to add *regulation* information to the structure, for example in order to tag restricted areas in a building,
- to identify objects, rooms, and zones;
- to represent connexity information;
- to add specific information to certain kinds of objects; for instance information about painters could be associated with sculptures in a museum.

Solutions – Linking Semantics to Structure Having stated the general problem above, we propose here our contributions and solutions. We introduce a particular means of representing semantic information, and linking it to the structure, using the model introduced in section 4.3.

We propose to represent semantic information using the Resource Description Framework (RDF) [27], an emerging W3C standard quite close to the theory of conceptual graphs [28]. We think that this choice makes sense because of the wide adoption of RDF by the industry. Thus, they are already a number applications able to handle RDF, and their number is steadily increasing.

In RDF, information is considered as a set of *assertions* that link objects of interest (sometimes called *resources*) together. Assertions are denoted by triples:

```
(subject, property, object)
```

An RDF description is composed of an arbitrary number of these triples, thus create multiple links between elements. This way, elements are connected in what is called an *RDF graph*.

Resources can be instances of classes. Several mechanisms have been proposed to describe class hierarchies. However, the *de facto* standard is OWL, which is the Web Ontology Language [29].

If we use RDF to represent semantic information, we end up with two worlds: one, a world of structure descriptions (possibly expressed in XML according to our model, described in section 4.3), and the other is a world of semantic annotations (expressed in RDF). These annotations exist only with respect to the underlying structure of buildings and they *need* to be connected to it.

To link semantic descriptions to the architectural elements of the structure description, we introduce a particular class of objects in the RDF descriptions. This is the class `Place`. Instances of `Place` correspond to architectural elements of the structure description and enable semantic graphs to be *anchored* in the structure. The actual correspondence is achieved through the use of a common identifier.

On figure 12, we can see the role played by the instances of class `Place`: these belong to the RDF graph, but they correspond one-to-one with the structural elements.

In practice, the structure in fig. 12 looks like this:

```
...
  <Building id="building-34">
    <Floor id="floor-1">
      <Office id="office-210">
        ...
      </Office>
    </Floor>
  </Building>
...
```

The triples of the associated semantic descriptions look like this:

```
(jack, hasCategory, crewMembers)
(crewMembers, hasAccessTo, privateAreas)
(jack, worksIn, office-210)
(floor-1, hasCategory, privateAreas)
...
(jack, rdf:type, Person)
(crewMembers, rdf:type, PersonelCategory)
(privateAreas, rdf:type, PlaceCategory)
(office-210, rdf:type, Place)
(floor-1, rdf:type, Place)
```

The structural elements `office-210` and `floor-1` have counterparts in the semantic description. The latter are instances of the class `Place`, and share the same identifier as their "structural" counterparts, which links the structure and semantics.

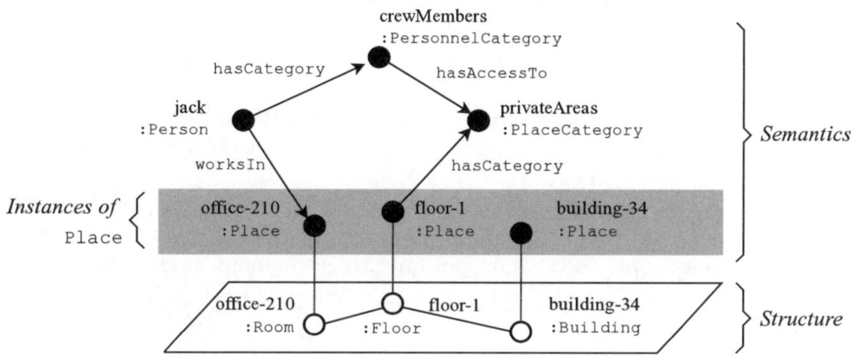

Fig. 12. Linking between semantics and structure.

Ontology for Semantic Annotations We have stated above that the objects of the RDF graphs are instances of classes and are defined using OWL. Here, we present some categories of objects that we think are important to include in an ontology for semantic annotations:

- *Locations:* in addition to the basic class `Place` already described, we propose a further two classes, `Function` that associates a function to a location (e.g. office, meeting room, etc.), and `PlaceCategory` that allows categories of places to be defined (with respect to an access restriction scheme, e.g. private area, public area, etc.);
- *People:* likewise, a class `Person` represents human beings, `Role` represents the roles played by people within an organization (e.g. employee, visitor, etc.), and `PersonnelCategory` allows categories of people to be specified. Again we use an access restriction scheme, staff member, intern, for example. It is not necessary to define a new class to represent persons. Instead, one can use the existing class `Person` from the FOAF (Friend Of A Friend) ontology [30];
- *Schedules:* to associate events to locations in a flexible way, we propose to define two classes: `Schedule` and `Event`.

The ontology may also define a whole set of RDF properties, used to specify relations between class instances. For example, `hasCategory` can be used to associate a `PersonnelCategory` to a `Person` or a `PlaceCategory` to a `Place`; `hasAccessTo` states that a `Person` or a `PersonnelCategory` have access to a `Place` or `PlaceCategory`.

Reasoning More than just enabling the description of complex relationships, a semantic description allows the definition of reasoning rules.

For instance, in the example of fig. 12 we have the following triples:

```
(jack, hasCategory, crewMembers)
(crewMembers, hasAccessTo, privateAreas)
(floor-1, hasCategory, privateAreas)
```

From that, it seems reasonable to deduce the additional triple:

```
(jack, hasAccessTo, floor-1)
```

Thanks to reasoning rules, it is possible to implement such *common sense* behaviors, and thus enable the automatic deduction of new triples from the set of existing ones.

5 Perspectives: Towards Ambient Intelligence

In 2001, Anind K. Dey defined the notion of *context* in human-computer interaction as *"any information that can be used to characterize the situation of entities [...] that are considered relevant to the interaction between a user and an application, including the user and the application themselves"* [31].

In this regard, the class of systems that we have presented here are *context-aware*. At the very least, their behavior, as well as the information they provide, depend on the location of the user. In reality, they could use many more aspects of context. For instance, taking ambient light into account provides useful information about activity in office buildings. For example when lights are off, employees are not likely to be at work.

Described as such, locomotion assistance devices would be applications for the numerous proposed frameworks for context-awareness, such as Anind K. Dey's own Context Toolkit [31] or Gaëtan Rey's Contextors [32]. They would be autonomous devices, constantly trying to extract contextual information from the surrounding environments, by reading physical sensors and querying data sources. This way, the environment is essentially unaware of the presence of blind users.

In contrast, we can imagine situations in which the environment is aware of the presence of users with special needs. For instance, if a door *knew* that a blind person is approaching, it could give hints through speech synthesis (*"Push to open!"*). Conversely, if a deaf person was approaching the door, it would not use speech synthesis, but rather flash a label with the word *"Push"* written on it.

In this case, information flows are much better than simple context-aware systems. Locomotion assistance devices behave as mobile *agents*, communicating with other agents embedded in the environment. This view corresponds to the notion of *ambient intelligence* [33] in which various objects have embedded computing capabilities as well as interaction facilities.

6 Conclusion

This chapter has described features, issues and solutions for next-generation mobility assistance devices for the blind. Figure 13 show an overview of what such a system could be, in terms of technological solutions.

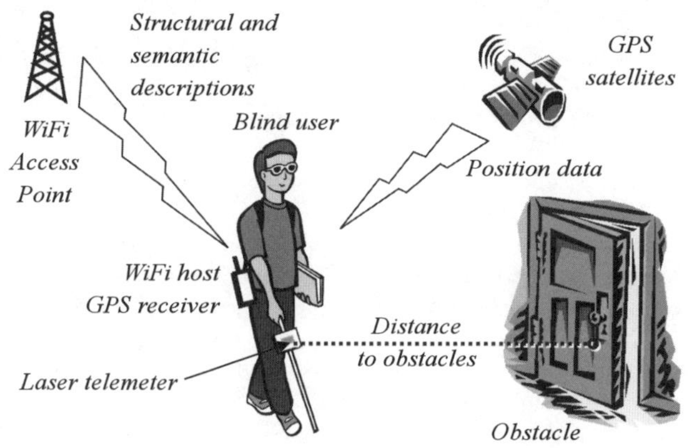

Fig. 13. Overview of a possible system.

This system builds upon existing electronic travel aids for the blind. It is based on a white cane, with a laser telemeter. However, it offers further features than just detecting close obstacles. Indeed, it permanently knows its position, thanks to a GPS receiver that works outside, and a WiFi positioning system that takes over the GPS inside buildings. Cartography and associated semantic descriptions are retrieved through the network, and provides guidance information as well as descriptive details about places.

This scheme remains relatively simple, because the handheld device communicates with its environment only to retrieve descriptions. However, a shift into ambient intelligence would turn the device into an *agent* communicating with various other agents located in the environment when the user visits new places.

The techniques needed by travel aids for the blind are not specific to this kind of applications. They can be applied to any context-aware mobile device, such as museum guide tours, travellers' assistants, and so forth.

References

1. Jansson, G.: The functions of present and future electronic travel aids for visually impaired children and adults. In The Spanish National Organization of the Blind, ed.: Sixth International Mobility Conference, (1991) 59–64
2. Blash, B.B., Long, R.G.: Use or non-use of electronic travel aids in the united states. In The Spanish National Organization of the Blind, ed.: Sixth International Mobility Conference, (1991) 49–58
3. Farcy, R., Denise, B., Damaschini, R.: Triangulating laser profilometer as a navigational aid for the blind: optical aspects. Applied Optics **35** (1996) 1161–1166
4. Farcy, R., Bellik, Y.: Comparison of various interface modalities for a locomotion assistance device. In Miesenberger, K., Klaus, J., Zagler, W., eds.: Computers Helping People with Special Needs, Springer (2002) 421–428
5. Farcy, R., Bellik, Y.: Locomotion assistance for the blind. In Keates, S., Langdom, P., Clarkson, P., Robinson, P., eds.: Universal Access and Assistive Technology, Springer (2002) 277–284
6. Baudoin, G., Venard, O., Uzan, G., Paumier, A., Cesbron, J.: Le projet RAMPE: système interactif d'information auditive pour la mobilité des personnes aveugles dans les transports publics. In: Proceedings of Ubimob 2005, Grenoble, France (2005) 169–176
7. Hightower, J., Borriello, G.: Location systems for ubiquitous computing. IEEE Computer **34** (2001) 57–66
8. Chao, J., Chen, Y., Wu Chen, X.D., Li, Z., Wong, N., Yu, M.: An Experimental Investigation into the Performance of GPS-based Vehicle Positioning in Very Dense Urban Areas. Journal of Geospatial Engineering **3** (2001) 59–66
9. Samama, N., Vervisch-Picois, A., Francois, M.: La localisation en intérieur à l'aide de répéteurs GPS: vers un système de positionnement universel ? In: Proceedings of Ubimob 2005, Grenoble, France (2005) 21–28
10. Anne, M., Crowley, J.L., Devin, V., Privat, G.: Localisation intra-bâtiment multi-technologies: RFID, wifi, vision. In: Proceedings of Ubimob 2005, Grenoble, France (2005) 29–35
11. Daniele, N., Pezzin, M., Derivaz, S., Keignart, J., Rouzet, P.: Principle and motivations of UWB technology for high data rate WPAN applications. In: Proceedings of sOc 2003, Grenoble, France (2003) 84–87
12. Schilit, B.N., Adams, N., Gold, R., Tso, M., Want, R.: The PARCTAB mobile computing system. In: Proceedings Fourth Workshop on Workstation Operating Systems (WWOS-IV), IEEE (1993) 34–39
13. Schilit, B., Adams, N., Want, R.: Context-aware computing applications. In: IEEE Workshop on Mobile Computing Systems and Applications, Santa Cruz, CA, US (1994) 85–90
14. Long, S., Kooper, R., Abowd, G.D., Atkeson, C.G.: Rapid prototyping of mobile context-aware applications: The cyberguide case study. In: Mobile Computing and Networking. (1996) 97–107
15. Römer, K., Schoch, T., Mattern, F., Dübendorfer, T.: Smart identification frameworks for ubiquitous computing applications. Wirel. Netw. **10** (2004) 689–700
16. Ni, L.M., Liu, Y., Lau, Y.C., Patil, A.P.: Landmarc: indoor location sensing using active rfid. Wirel. Netw. **10** (2004) 701–710
17. Hähnel, D., Burgard, W., Fox, D., Fishkin, K., Philipose, M.: Mapping and localization with RFID technology. In: Proc. of the IEEE International Conference on Robotics and Automation (ICRA). (2004) 1015–1020

18. Floerkemeier, C., Lampe, M.: Issues with rfid usage in ubiquitous computing applications. In Ferscha, A., Mattern, F., eds.: Pervasive Computing: Second International Conference, PERVASIVE 2004. Number 3001 in LNCS, Linz/Vienna, Austria, Springer-Verlag (2004) 188–193
19. Brusey, J., Floerkemeier, C., Harrison, M., Fletcher, M.: Reasoning about uncertainty in location identification with rfid. Workshop on Reasoning with Uncertainty in Robotics at IJCAI (2003)
20. LaMarca, A., Chawathe, Y., Consolvo, S., Hightower, J., Smith, I., Scott, J., Sohn, T., Howard, J., Hughes, J., Potter, F., Tabert, J., Powledge, P., Borriello, G., Schilit, B.: Place lab: Device positioning using radio beacons in the wild. In: Proceedings of the 3rd International Conference on Pervasive Computing (Pervasive 2005). Volume 3468 of LNCS., Springer-Verlag (2005)
21. Krumm, J., Cermak, G., Horvitz, E.: Rightspot: A novel sense of location for a smart personal object. In Dey, A.K., Schmidt, A., McCarthy, J.F., eds.: UbiComp 2003: Ubiquitous Computing, 5th International Conference, Seattle, WA, USA, October 12-15, 2003, Proceedings. Volume 2864 of Lecture Notes in Computer Science., Springer (2003) 36–43
22. Fusiello, A., Caprile, B.: Synthesis of Indoor Maps in Presence of Uncertainty. Robotics and Autonomous Systems **22** (1997) 103–114
23. Kitazawa, K., Konishi, Y., Shibasaki, R.: A Method of Map Matching For Personal Positioning Systems. In: Proceedings of the Asian Conference on Remote Sensing ACRS 2000, (2000) 726–731
24. Web 3D Consortium: The Virtual Reality Modeling Language International Standard ISO/IEC 14772-1:1997. Technical report, Web 3D Consortium (1997) Available at `http://www.web3d.org/x3d/specifications/vrml/ISO-IEC-14772-IS-VRML97WithAmendment1/`.
25. Web 3D Consortium: Extensible 3D (X3D) International Standard ISO/IEC FCD 19775:200x Final Committee Draft. Technical report, Web 3D Consortium (2003) Available at `http://www.web3d.org/x3d/specifications/x3d_specification.html`.
26. Hadzilacos, T., Tryfona, N.: An extended entity-relationship model for geographic applications. SIGMOD Record **26** (1997) 24–29
27. Manola, F., Miller, E., McBride, B.: RDF primer. Technical report, W3C World Wide Web Consortium (2003)
28. Sowa, J.F.: Conceptual graphs for a database interface. IBM Journal of Research and Development **20** (1976) 336–357
29. McGuinness, D.L., van Harmelen, F.: OWL web ontology language overview. Technical report, W3C World Wide Web Consortium (2003)
30. Dumbill, E.: Finding friends with XML and RDF. `http://www-106.ibm.com/developerworks/xml/library/x-foaf.html` (2002)
31. Dey, A.K., Salber, D., Abowd, G.: A conceptual framework and a toolkit for supporting the rapid prototyping of context-aware applications. Human Computer Interaction **16** (2001) 97–166
32. Coutaz, J., Rey, G.: Foundations for a theory of contextors. In: Computer-Aided Design of User Interfaces III, Proceedings of the Fourth International Conference on Computer-Aided Design of User Interfaces, Kluwer (2002) 13–34
33. Ducatel, K., Bogdanowicz, M., Scapolo, F., Leijten, J., Burgelman, J.C.: Scenarios for ambient intelligence in 2010. Final report, IST Advisory Group (ISTAG), European Commission (2001)

6. Multimedia Communication System for the Blind

Makoto Kobayashi[1] and Tetsuya Watanabe[2]

[1] Department of Computer Science, Tsukuba College of Technology, Kasuga 4-12-7, Tsukuba City, Ibaraki, Japan
koba@cs.k.tsukuba-tech.ac.jp
http://www.cs.k.tsukuba-tech.ac.jp/labo/koba

[2] National Institute of Special Education, Nobi 5-1-1, Yokosuka City, Kanagawa, Japan
twatanab@nise.go.jp
http://www.nise.go.jp/research/kogaku/twatanab/indexEn.html

Abstract. A Multimedia communication system for blind users is developed. The system is named MIMIZU and its terminal is composed of a refreshable tactile graphic display and a stylus pen device that utilizes ultrasonic technologies. Blind users can make drawings directly on the tactile display surface with the stylus pen. It was originally developed as a drawing system with an erasing function. As the research progresses, we have noticed that it has a potential as a communication system for the blind with multimedia interactions. To implement the system, we made a pair of terminals and connected them by a network cable and developed communication software for a whiteboard application. Using the system, a pair of blind users can make and share tactile image information with each other. We describe results of a simple experiment in which one subject tried to transmit simple drawings to the other subject using this system. The tactile display's resolution presented the difficulty in transmitting a circle, but the results were useful when transmitting shapes based on straight lines. Even when the subject is a circle, it is recognized when prior information is available. In addition to the communication software, we developed a type of ping-pong game for the system. The ball is shown by four pins arranged in a square and it moves from side to side. To play the game, players must hit the ball with a racket controlled by the stylus pen. The experiment with blind players showed that they could enjoy this game.

M. Kobayashi and T. Watanabe: *Multimedia Communication System for the Blind*, Studies in Computational Intelligence (SCI) **19**, 165–181 (2006)
www.springerlink.com

1. Introduction

It is important for the blind to know and understand graphical information using their tactile sense. To acquire this information, they usually use tangible or tactile materials such as embossed pictures, drawings on swellpaper or reliefs on foil. Undoubtedly these tangible materials are useful for them to understand spatial information. Early research showed that subjects could do a simple matching task between tangible pictures even if they had no visual experience [1]. It seems that the act of drawing is not common in the daily life of blind people. In spite of that they can use graphical information and there are drawing tools available for them such as raised-line drawing kits. We think one of the drawbacks is that those tools do not allow the blind user to erase raised lines. With this background, we began a project to develop an "erasable" drawing system for the blind.

We can cite TDraw [2] as a preceding research project. This was one of the drawing systems developed for the blind. It was composed using a thermo pen and swellpaper on a digitizer that detects position of the thermo pen. TDraw was not an erasable system because it mainly aimed to record how the blind subjects make drawings and to analyze the mental model they have. Hence the system did not need to have a function to erase. Our standpoint was different to this. We mainly focused on the problem of erasing raised lines for more flexible drawing.

2. History of MIMIZU

Several months after our project started, a prototype system was developed in 2000[1]. From the beginning of the project, we had assumed that the system should be composed of refreshable tactile graphic display units and a stylus pen because refreshable display units are the only way to make tactile information erasable. In realizing this system, a problem was how to detect the position of the stylus pen over the tactile display units that have actuators and pins underneath. There was no space to align positioning sensors on the display. Our solution to the problem was very simple: connecting a stylus pen with beam arms and setting angular sensors between the arms. With this architecture, a computer can calculate the position of the stylus pen tip from the length of the beam arms and angular information between these arms. The moving range of the pen was bounded by the arms but it worked well and achieved the first goal. We named the system MIMIZU, which means a kind of worm in Japan. The motion of the tactile display pins is similar to that of the worm.

The workflow of the prototype system was as follows. When the program starts, the computer waits for the user's action. If the user moves the stylus pen over the tactile graphic display with the drawing-button on the pen pressed, the computer calculates the position of the pen tip and raises the tactile pins under the pen tip. If the user moves the stylus with the erasing-button pressed, the tactile pins under the pen tip are lowered. If the user presses the clear button, all of the tactile pins are lowered. While the user presses any one of these buttons, the computer plays a certain sound that differs depending on the button pressed. This sound information helps the blind user to recognize which operation they are doing at that moment. In this way, the user can make drawings and erase arbitrary parts of the drawings. Also the drawing image can be saved as an electronic file on the computer and reloaded later.

Furthermore, the program has an animation function. With this function, the user can make tactile drawings blink or move from the right side to the left or left to right. This animated tactile drawing can also be displayed against the background of a fixed drawing. For example, two fixed axes expressed as crossed lines at right angles and a moving sine curve can be displayed simultaneously. A blinking animation function makes the main foreground drawing easily distinguishable from the fixed background drawing. The blind user can easily recognize a blinking foreground tactile image against the fixed background.

Since we made the first prototype system, we have continued to improve. Fig.1 shows MIMIZU developed in 2002[4]. It was equipped with a wireless LCD tablet to provide for easy input. By using the tablet, a sighted user can make a drawing directly on the tablet with either of a pen or a finger, and a blind user can touch and recognize the drawing which appears on the tactile graphic display. The blind user also can add more lines it or erase part of the drawing.

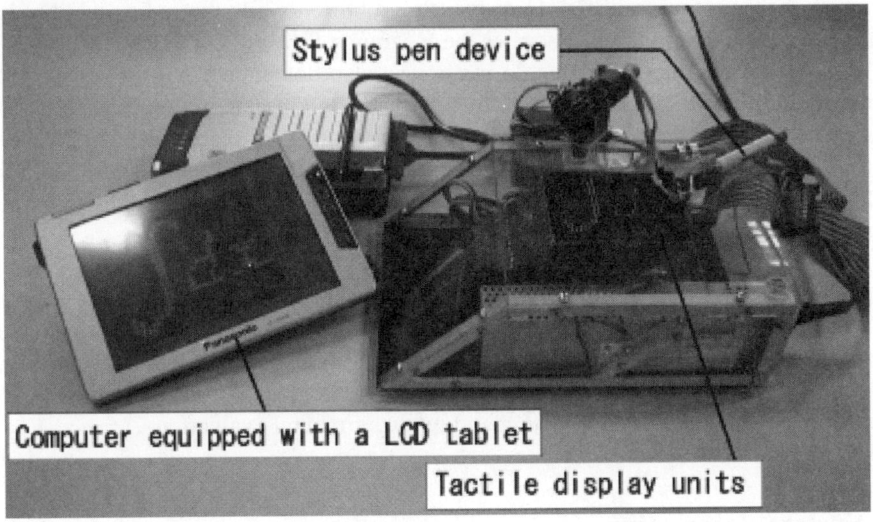

Fig. 1. An overview of the MIMIZU system in 2002. It was composed of a stylus pen device connected with beam arms and angular sensors, a computer which was equipped with a wireless LCD tablet, and tactile display units served as a matrix

In parallel with the improvement of hardware, we made some software programs for MIMIZU. After making the drawing and animation programs mentioned above, realized that our hardware components are usable as an interactive multimedia system for the blind also. This system allows the blind user to input position information directly on the tactile surface and to receive feedback of changing tactile information or by sound information.

Based on this viewpoint, a ping-pong game was developed. In this game, a player has to pursue a ball expressed by four tactile pins by touching it with fingers, and to strike it back by a racket expressed as a short tactile line. The player controls the position of the racket using the stylus pen. The ball moves a straight line and bounces off the walls of the top, bottom, and left side. The racket is set at the right side, and is allowed to move only in the vertical direction. When the ball bounces off the wall or is hit by the racket, a knocking sound is played. This game is very simple and easy to play if you can see the display monitor, however, it is difficult to play when using only with the tactile sense.

After developing this game, we made some Kanji learning software. Most Kanji characters are built of several "bushu" radicals each of which has different meanings. Usually we use tangible educational materials to teach Kanji characters to students in special schools for the blind. Even so, it is difficult to distinguish these components only by touching them. To solve the problem, we used the blinking animation and sound feedback functions. When a blind user moves the stylus pen over any radical of a Kanji character that is displayed on the tactile surface, the radical starts to blink. It helps the user to recognize the shape of the radical and distinguish it from other radicals. Also, pressing a button while the radical is blinking generates speech output that describes the meaning of the radical more precisely.

A program for interactive tactile maps was also developed. A user can acquire detailed auditory description of an arbitrary place on the map by pointing to it with the stylus with the button pressed. Moreover, using this software when another button is zoom up and zoom down functions are available. By pressing the zoom up button, the tactile display shows a more detailed map around where the stylus pen points.

Soon after these improvements to hardware and software, a pen device which can input information to a computer using ultrasonic technology came on the market. We decided to use the technology for MIMIZU instead of the stylus pen connected to beam arms. We tried to use MIMIZU as a communication system for the blind users by connecting a pair of terminals with a network cable. In following section we describe detail of the new system and its experimental evaluation.

3. System description

The MIMIZU is basically composed of a refreshable tactile graphic display, an input device, and a computer which controls these devices. Fig. 2 shows an overview of the terminal of MIMIZU with an ultrasonic pen on use. A pair of such terminals were connected by a network cable.

3.1 Tactile graphic display

The area of the tactile graphic display is double that of the earlier version of MIMIZU. It measures 144mm by 96mm, and includes 1536 pins arranged in a matrix of 48 pins in the columns and 32 pins in rows. The inter-pin spaces are 3 mm, and the pin stroke is about 1mm. The principle of driving those pins is the same as common refreshable Braille displays and by using piezoelectric actuators. By applying high voltage electricity the stick-shaped actuators bend and raise the tactile pins. The actuators are controlled by an LSI unit which receives controlling signals from the computer. Fig. 3 shows an overview and the principle of SC-5, the tactile display unit that we used as the components of the tactile surface.

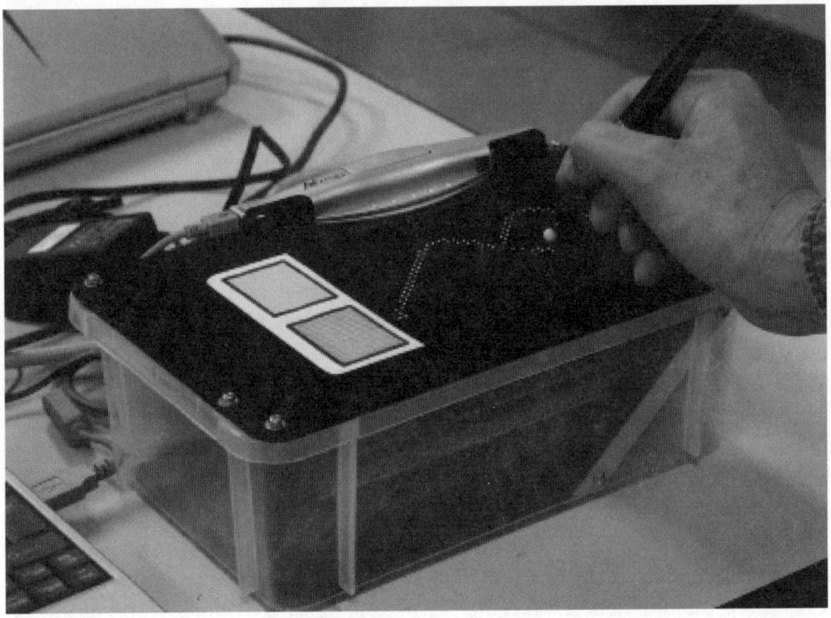

Fig. 2. An overview of a MIMIZU terminal equipped with an ultrasonic pen. It is composed of a refreshable tactile graphic display, an ultrasonic stylus pen device, and a computer. While the whiteboard programs are running, the user can make a drawing on the display with the stylus pen and the same drawing appears on the receiving terminal. In the match-up ping pong game, the players control their racket by means of the stylus pen

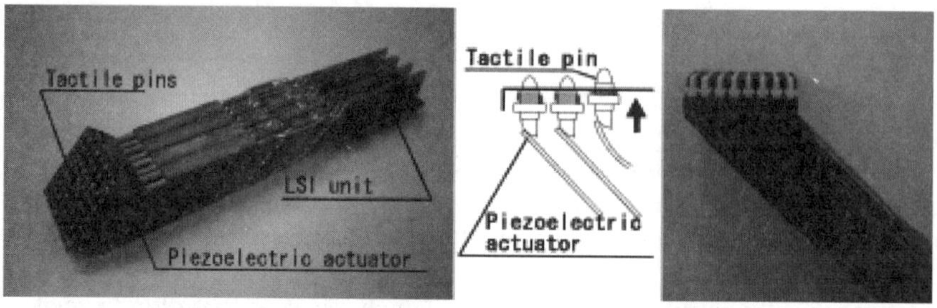

Fig. 3. Left: an overview of SC-5, the tactile graphic display unit. Middle: the principle of driving pins by bending piezoelectric actuators. Right: the side view of SC-5 without the top cover

3.2 Stylus pen utilizing ultrasonic technology

Applying ultrasonic technology by using the stylus pen is the main improvement in this version of MIMIZU. The measurement principle is as follows. The stylus pen has a micro switch and transducers for ultrasonic and infrared at its tip. The stylus pen includes batteries in its body. The receiver unit, when applied to the upper side of the tactile surface, has two receivers which detect both signals. When the user presses the stylus pen onto the tactile surface, the transducers on the pen tip emit ultrasonic and infrared signals. Each receiver then detects the distance from the pen tip to the receivers using the time between the two signals. The receivers then calculate the position of the tip of the stylus by the triangulation method. The positioning resolution is 1200 points per inch. The advantage of using this device is its spatial flexibility. The stylus pen is not bound to the body of the system. The user can use several terminals, without changing the styli. We have noticed a disadvantage that the user must pay attention and not obstruct the pen tip during manipulation. If the user does, the signals from the pen tip will be stopped from reaching the receivers. That is, when the user lets his fingers follow the pen tip to support the motion of the pen, he must keep his fingers away from path between the pen tip and the receivers. This is a problem for a sighted user. It requires practice for the blind user to use stylus in this way.

3.3 Functional scheme of whiteboard application

As a trial application for the new hardware, we used a whiteboard application. The aim is to establish communication of drawings between two blind users. The basic scheme of each terminal is almost same as in the first MIMIZU. The computer waits for user's action and then controls the pins under the pen tip. Raising them if the user wants them to be part of the drawing and lowering them if he wants to erase. The ultrasonic pen has no buttons unlike the stylus pen of the first system.

We designed the new system which has two states, the drawing and the erasing mode. Users can change these modes by tapping the designated square area with the ultrasonic pen. The tapping area is on the left side of the tactile surface (See Fig. 2) and blind users can detect that area as it has a unique texture. Adjacent to this area, there is another square area that has a different texture for clear all pins. If the user taps this area, all tactile pins are lowered. To help the user to confirm each action, different sound files are played as in the first system.

With this scheme, users can make drawings on each tactile surface. During the drawing operations, the same graphic appears on the tactile display of the other terminal. They share the same graphic information.

3.4 Functional scheme of match-up type ping-pong game

After the development of the whiteboard application, we made match-up type ping-pong game for an entertainment purposes. When the game starts, a player has to pursue a moving ball expressed by four tactile pins, and he has to strike it back by a racket using the stylus pen in the same way as in the former system. The ball speed as determined by the computer moves the ball by 3mm every 150msec. Consequently, it takes about eight seconds for the ball to travel from one side to the other. The traveling time varies depending on the angle of the path. This game is different from the first game in two ways. Firstly, a player competes against the other human player instead of playing the computer. The upside-down image is simultaneously displayed on the other tactile terminal. Secondly, the player is allowed to move his racket anywhere in the tactile surface. The player does not know when the other player returned the ball because the player's racket doesn't appear on their display. Fig. 4 shows sequential images of how the game is played and how it appears on the tactile display. The game was designed only for a right-handed player.

4. Experiment of transmitting images using whiteboard software

The first experiment was done to evaluate the whiteboard software. We designed the software to allow blind users to make interactive communication with it. It means that users can understand and modify the images that the opponents have drawn on their own terminal. As a first step, we need to know how correctly the images can be transmitted from one user to the other user. We made a simple experiment similar to a "telephone game" in which the system conveys tactile drawings instead of speech. By comparing the reproduced drawings, we evaluated the system.

4.1 Participants

A pair of blind students participated in the experiment. Both of them were Braille readers and claimed to have normal tactile sense. They usually used tactile materials to get information for their studies. Subject A was male and lost his sight due to orbital tumor when he was born. He has a little light perception with the right eye, but could not distinguish the number of displayed fingers in front of his face. Subject B was female and was totally, congenitally blind due to enucleation of eyeball with retinoblastoma. Both subjects were twenty years old at the time of the experiment.

4.2 Experimental procedure

A pair of MIMIZU terminals were connected by a network cable, and a whiteboard was installed. We prepared four types of line drawings printed on swellpaper. Each sheet of swellpaper had two simple figures on it. They were presented in two directions; one side up the first time and facing down the second time. In total eight kinds of target pictures were presented to the subjects. To record the handwritten results made by the subjects, we prepared raised-line drawing kits. A tangible square rim represents the area for drawing was made on every vinyl sheet in advance.

Prior to performing the above experiment mentioned, subjects were informed of the functions and usage of the MIMIZU system. The procedure of the experiment was then discussed. The kind of tactile images which would be presented was not disclosed.

The experiment was the composed of two sets. In the first set, four trials were conducted using four different target pictures. Subject A was required to send the image to Subject B. The main flow of the first set is shown in the Fig. 5. In the second set, the roles were changed. This time, the target pictures were presented upside down.

In each trial firstly, one subject the "sender" was required to recognize a target picture by touching it. Then, the sender then made a drawing using a MIMIZU terminal. The other subject who was a "receiver" felt the tactile image on the other terminal while the sender was drawing. The receiver then made a drawing using a raised-line drawing kit and a ballpoint pen to show what he felt. During the trials subjects were not allowed to talk to each other about the shapes of drawings, so the results could only come from tactile information.

It was difficult to remove an effect of each subjects' tactile sensitivity and drawing skill. To account for this effect, both subjects were required to make drawings on swellpaper immediately after feeling the original target pictures at the end of each set of the experiment. We can consider the effect by comparing all of the images drawn.

Every experiment was recorded by two digital video cameras to record the behavior of the subjects.

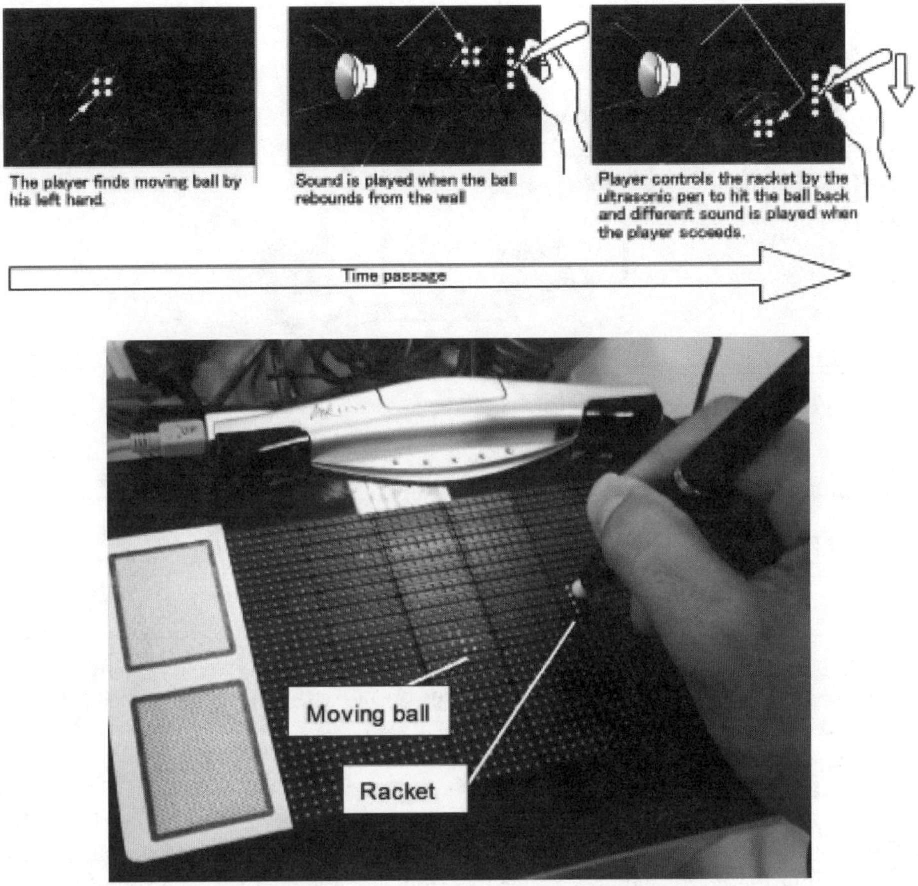

Fig. 4. Upper: sequential images of how the player plays the ping-pong game. The player pursues the moving ball by left hand and controls the racket pins with the ultrasonic pen held by the right hand. He has to anticipate the motion of the ball and hit it back in another direction. Lower: how the tactile surface displays the ball and the racket

4.3 Results

Fig. 6 shows eight pairs of prepared target pictures printed on swellpaper and the final drawings made by the receiver using raised-line drawing kit. The left four pairs show the results of the first set; when the pictures were transmitted from Subject A to Subject B. The right four pairs are those of the second set when the transmission was from Subject B to Subject A.

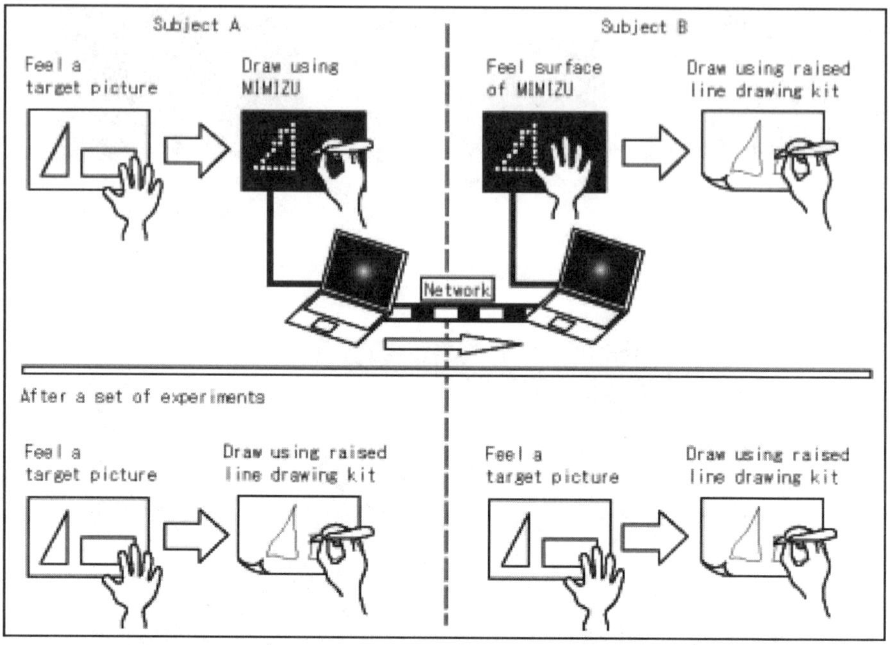

Fig. 5. Experimental procedure. The "sender" draws an image on a MIMIZU terminal after touching a target picture. The "receiver" feels the image which the sender draws and, then, reproduces the image using a raised-line drawing kit

4.4 Discussion

The four drawings in the right column in Fig. 6, results of the second set, seem to be reproducing the target pictures better than those of the first set. We found that the main difference between these sets is the reproduction of the circle. It is said that drawing a circle without visual sense is very difficult. Subject A commented the same after the experiment. Additionally, we think that the resolution problem of the tactile display has a strong effect. Dot matrix approximation with inter-pin spaces of 3 mm is not fine enough to curved lines such as a circle. Those two results made us to speculate that Subject B recognized the circle as a small square and her comment after the experiment supported this speculation. She thought the line as straight because the circle that Subject A drew was composed of a few short lines. Why were the circles in the second set were reproduced better? We think the difference of conditions between the first and second set accounted for the difference of the results. In the second set, the receiver Subject A already had some knowledge of what kind of pictures would appear on the tactile surface. He could have anticipated the shapes. We compared the circle images which appeared on tactile surface, and they were not very different in shape. It means that advanced knowledge helped to produce correct drawings. We can say that proper advanced information helps to produce a better image.

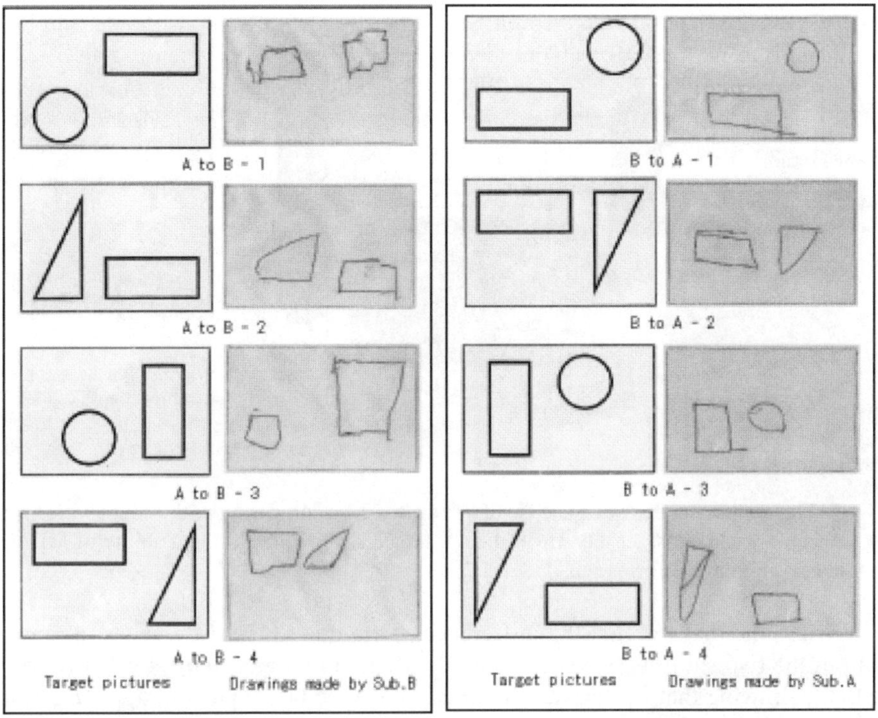

Fig. 6. Eight kinds of target pictures printed on swellpaper and the answers drawn by the "receiver" subject. The left four cases are the results obtained in the first set. Hence, images were transmitted from Subject A to Subject B. The right four cases are those of the second set; where images were transmitted from Subject B to Subject A.

To obtain more detailed analysis of the trials, we made the analyzing chart shown in Fig.7. It is an example of the trial of "A to B - 2" in Fig.6. The upper left figure is the target picture. The lower left is the drawing made by the sender after touching the target picture. The figure in the center is the drawing made by Subject A on the tactile surface of MIMIZU. The same tactile image as this appeared on the terminal in front of the Subject B. The upper right figure is the drawing made by Subject B just after touching the target picture. The lower right figure is the drawing made by Subject B after touching the drawing on the tactile display terminal, the same as the drawing in the center.

In this chart we can find a few differences between the target picture on the upper left, and the Subject B's final drawing on the lower right. (1) The height of the left triangle is less than the target picture. (2) The baselines of the two objects are at different levels although they are the same as in the target picture. (3) The right rectangle of the final drawing has a little bump at its upper line. (4) The left corner of the left triangle is rounded in the final drawing.

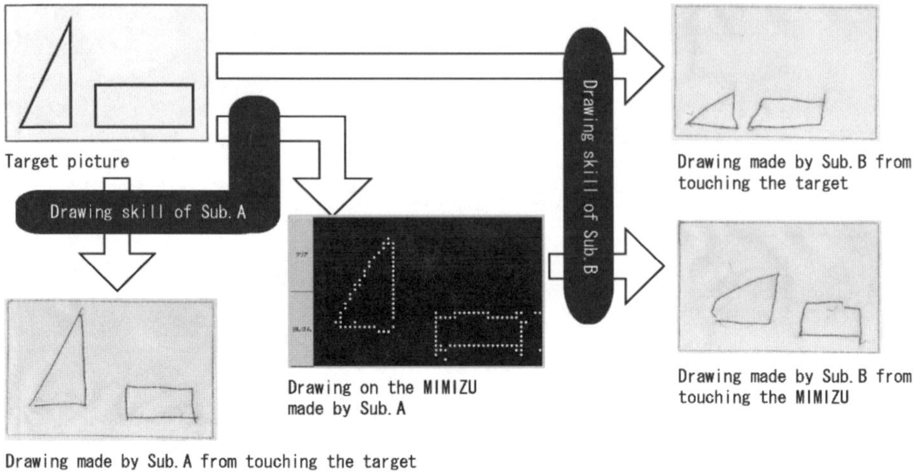

Fig. 7. The analyzing chart of the case of "A to B – 2." Comparing with the drawings made by subject, we can consider the effect of each subjects' drawing skill and ability of MIMIZU to transmit an image information

We assume that the first two differences were due to the differences in drawing skill of the two subjects. If we compare the final drawing of Subject B (lower right) with the drawing that is reproduced directly from the target picture, upper right, it is clear that Subject B has a tendency to draw a triangle smaller than the original one and that Subject A has a tendency to draw baselines at different levels. Regarding last two differences, we think they were due to the characteristics of the system, mainly the tactile images expressed by a dot matrix. Firstly, it is difficult to draw straight lines on the tactile surface of the system. Consequently, the upper line of the rectangle drawn by Subject A on the tactile display had a little bump. Secondly, this bump is perceived as a big one by touch although it is small when perceived by vision. The rounded edge of the triangle is also explained by the difference between touch and vision. We can perceive the left triangle in the drawing on the tactile display as a triangle if we see the whole figure. Then, we would ignore the fact that the detailed shape of its lower corner is not clearly cut. However, if we feel it with fingers, the corner is felt as rounded.

In the future work, we should add a new function of helping the user to draw straight lines, which is common drawing software for sighted users. Also we have to find or develop technologies which can improve the input device and realize higher resolution of the tactile display.

5. Evaluation of a match-up type ping-pong game

We next tried to evaluate the match-up type ping-pong game. Generally evaluation of entertainment systems is difficult. Because of this, we only required subjects to describe impressions and comments about the game after a few minutes of trial use. We also recorded their behaviors by a digital video camera. In this section, these impressions and behavior are described and discussed.

5.1 Participants

Two pairs of blind students participated in the session voluntarily. The members of the first pair were the same students who participated in the prior experiment, Subjects A and Subject B. Additionally two participants, Subjects C and D took part in this evaluation. Both were Braille readers and had normal tactile sense. They also usually used tactile materials to get information in their study and used screen readers to operate the computer. Subject C was male and had glaucoma. He has residual sight in his right eye, but no sight in his left eye. Subject D was also male and he became visually impaired in the age of thirteen due to craniopharyngioma. He can count the number of fingers held in front of his face with the right eye, but not with the left eye. These subjects were eighteen at the time of the experiment.

5.2 Experimental procedure

After explaining the system components and usage of the game subjects were requested to play the game more than five minutes of time. Fig.8 is a snapshot taken while Subject C and D were playing the game. After playing the game, the subjects were asked to frankly describe their impressions and comments about the game.

5.3 Results and Discussion

The video film recording showed that all the subjects successfully played the game. Subject B were not able to find the moving ball at first. In five minutes, she became used to the manipulation and able to hit the ball back by operating her racket by the ultrasonic pen. We consider the proposed game is not too difficult for the blind players. The pair of Subject C and D tried to play a high speed version and could enjoy it. In that version, the ball was moved by one pin every 100 msec; which is 1.5 times faster than the normal mode. Considering difficulty of the tactile game, Subject C commented as follows:

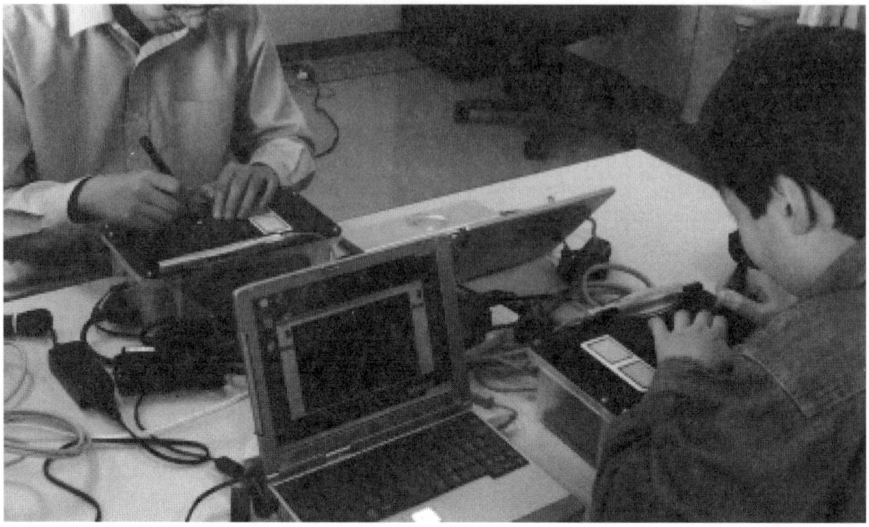

Fig. 8. Subjects C and D playing the match-up type ping-pong game by controlling the racket. Each terminal displays the moving ball only and the racket of the user of that terminal. The opponents racket is not displayed on their screen.

> "We could enjoy the high speed version, but a high speed game would not be enjoyable. It makes the game too hard to understand. An idea I have is to allow players to put obstacles on the court. Too much tactile information will be confusing to us and such an addition would require careful consideration."

This comment illustrated the difficulty in designing games with tactile display devices. Unlike home video games, tactile displays cannot express color and thickness information. It can only display a Boolean value. That is raised or lowered. We have to understand its this characteristic and pay particular attention to make distinguishable tactile components when adding more information to increase difficulty of the game. Utilizing real tactile material instead of raised tactile pins is one of the solutions. Following comments made by Subject C and D suggest the use of tactile materials.

- "It will become more interesting if you make the shape of the pen tip like a real racket."
- "How about putting a net line in the middle of the court? A physical wire would be helpful for a blind player."

These ideas are interesting to us. Home video games use many kinds of input and feedback devices. They use not only legacy devices such as joysticks, steering wheels, and pedals, but also musical instruments and other equipments such as violins, drums, and baseball bats. These devices have proper interfaces to play the game and easy to understand their use as they are real objects. Our tactile game for the blind player also should in the future have such good interfaces. Additionally, several subjects gave intriguing comments about the area of the tactile display.

- "If you provide a larger tactile area with the same density of tactile pins, it would not be suitable for the tactile game like this. If the purpose is limited to exploring some image information, it would be OK. Tactile games require speedy reaction, so users have to recognize all the information at a *touch*. From that viewpoint, a higher resolution of the tactile display is desirable. The tactile display area of this device is adequate."

We can conclude that too large tactile surfaces are not suitable for speedy interactive games.

We would like to quote the comments from all the subjects.

- "It was great fun. I want to play different kinds of games next time. Could you make another one?"

We were encouraged by the comment. We are now aware of the importance of tactile displays for entertainment.

6. Summary and further work

We developed MIMIZU, a multimedia communication system for the blind. The system is composed of a pair of terminals which is equipped with tactile display units and an ultrasonic pen. As applications of the system, we developed whiteboard software and match-up type ping-pong game. The evaluation by blind subjects showed that using this equipment they can transmit simple geometric figures and share the graphical information. However, the resolution problem of the tactile display surface still remains. Regarding the tactile game, it was shown that they enjoy it and have made valuable comments for the future design and improvement of tactile games using the tactile displays.

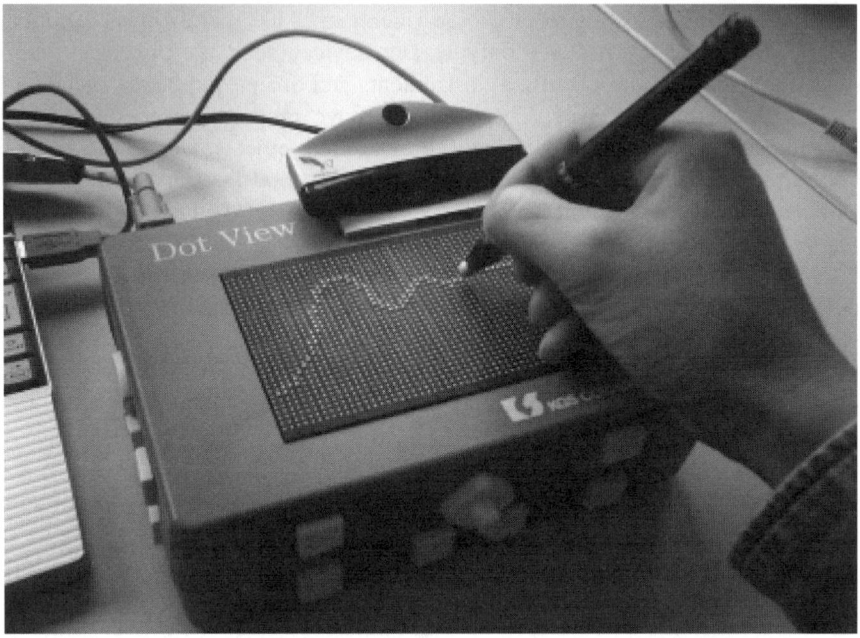

Fig. 9. We can now make MIMIZU in a consumer suitable tactile graphic display

A consumer version of tactile graphic display equipped with twelve tactile display units, SC-5, was put on the market in the autumn of 2002 by the Japanese company, KGS Corporation. Following our development and evaluation described above, the same company started to sell a new version of tactile graphic display in the spring of 2004. It has 1536 pins. The same number as in our system. The intervals of pins are 2.4 mm. Thanks to the product, people can purchase all the hardware components of MIMIZU. We no longer have to consume time to assemble hardware anymore. Fig. 9 shows the latest MIMIZU using the consumer version of tactile display. For future work, our research theme on tactile displays will be moved to development of useful software and its evaluation. We hope that more blind people will use our system and obtain enjoyment from it in the future.

Acknowledgement:

This research was partially supported by the Ministry of Education, Science, Sports and Culture, Grant-in-Aid for Scientific Research, 13680264(2001-2002), 15500400(2003-2004), and the Telecommunications Advancement Foundation(2001).

References

1. Heller, A., M., Brckett, D., D., and Scroggs, E.: Tangible Picture Matching by People Who Are Visually Impaired, Journal of Visual Impairment & Blindness, May, (2002) 349-353
2. Kurze, M.: TDraw: A Computer-based Tactile Drawing Tool for Blind People, ASSETS'96, Vancouver, (1996) 131-138
3. Watanabe, T. and Kobayashi, M.: A Prototype of the Freely Rewritable Tactile Drawing System for Perosons Who Are Blind, Journal of Visual Impairment & Blindness, (2002) 460-464
4. Kobayashi, M. and Watanabe, T.: A Tactile Display System Equipped with a Pointing Device –MIMIZU-, Computers Helping People with Special Needs, 8th ICCHP2002, Springer-Verlag (2002) 527-534

7 Information Technology for Deaf People

Marlene Hilzensauer

Center for Sign Language and Deaf Communication, University of Klagenfurt, Universitaetsstrasse 65-67, 9020 Klagenfurt, Austria
marlene.hilzensauer@uni-klu.ac.at

Abstract. In our modern information and communication society, daily life would be unthinkable without technology. Information and Communications Technology (ICT) is also very useful for people with special needs. As the acoustic channel is barred to the deaf, all acoustic data have to be presented in visual form, ideally in sign language. This chapter presents a general overview of the use of ICT for deaf people using current as well as future technologies. The focus is on communication, e-learning and barrier-free access to information. Various projects of the Center for Sign Language serve as practical examples, and illustrate the Austrian situation.

1 Introduction

New assistive technologies have helped many people to lead more comfortable lives. However, modern information and communications technology (ICT) is especially important for people with special needs. As the Communications Committee of the European Union so succinctly puts it:

> ICT plays a key role in the daily activities of any person. Whether it is employment, education, leisure, or at home. ICT is present in the form of computers, telephones and TV equipment. With the development of technology and the convergence of new platforms, these devices will play an increasing role in our daily activities. Many new and complex services are being offered through them. Access for people with disabilities to the Information Society is crucial for their integration and participation and their development as citizens with equal rights. [1]

Deaf people are at an additional disadvantage, because their handicap is practically 'invisible' from the outside with the exception of visible cochlear implants or hearing-aids. The public understand that people who cannot walk need a wheelchair or that blind people need Braille, but the need of the deaf for their native language as a sign language, is often overlooked. ICT can help here, especially with regard to multimedia technology, broadband connections and video capacities.

M. Hilzensauer: *Information Technology for Deaf People*, Studies in Computational Intelligence (SCI) **19**, 183–206 (2006)
www.springerlink.com

2 Sign Language

2.1 Sign Language as a Visual Language

As deaf people cannot hear, over the centuries they have developed another mode of communication that suits their unique needs and abilities. Sign languages use the visual channel - the signs are formed with special handshapes and movements and are produced in front of or placed on certain parts of the body (above the waist only). Formerly often regarded as simple 'pictures in the air', sign language is even today not officially recognized as a language in its own right in every country. In Austria, for instance, it was recognized only this year, because minority languages were defined ethnically.

Many hearing people are still of the opinion that sign language is only an auxiliary language, translating each word of a spoken language into a single sign. Although such auxiliary languages do exist (e.g. Signed English, Signed German/Lautsprachbegleitendes Gebaerden, etc.), real sign language is something entirely different. Contrary to popular belief, there is not only a single sign language common to all the deaf worldwide, but every country has its own sign language, even way different dialects - the same way as with spoken languages.

These national sign languages are real languages with their own grammar, sometimes radically different from spoken languages. For instance, sign languages make use of space as a grammatical element, due to their production in space. When signing how two cars crash into each other, you can show exactly how and where the two cars collide. Form is also very important: for instance, when signing how a door is opened, you can show your conversation partner whether the door is opened with a European handle or an American knob or whether it is an Asian sliding door. Frequently, a single sign can express a meaning for which you would need a whole sentence in a spoken language. This holds especially for the so-called classifiers which are excellent introductions to sign language and classifiers, see [2] and [3].

2.2. The Need for Sign Language

Hearing people are unfamiliar with deaf people's need for sign language. They think that if you cannot hear, you can easily access any necessary information by simply reading it in written form, and if you really need to communicate, you can always write your message down. There are some difficulties, however.

First, due to old-fashioned education methods relying almost exclusively on oral education which do not take into account their special needs. Consequently many of the deaf have only limited reading and writing skills:

> As a result, they are not only cut off from acoustically offered information but often also from written information. This is the reason why many sign language users need help with written language in spite of the fact that it is already available in the visual mode [4].

This is still true for Austria, for instance although this may hopefully change in the future. Many deaf people balk at longer or more difficult texts, and when writing themselves, they usually make grammatical mistakes which, in turn, cause them to avoid writing as much as possible. In order to understand something fully, they need it explained in sign language.

Secondly, because of its inherent qualities as a visual language, sign language is very hard to write down. For quickly noting sign language texts, glosses are commonly used. These are usually words taken from the national spoken language which correspond more or less to a sign. There are several problems with glosses, though: While some glosses are easy (e.g. CAT for the sign for 'cat'), many signs do not correlate with a single word; moreover, you need to know the sign beforehand, because reconstructing it from the gloss is impossible.

There are some scientific notations like the Stokoe-System [5] or HamNoSys [6] which describe how a certain sign is formed, but they are rather difficult to learn and are therefore used mostly by sign language researchers. There is one notable exception called SignWriting [7] was developed as a kind of everyday script for sign language. Although it is in widespread use in some countries like the USA, most of the Austrian deaf are not really familiar with it [1].

This is where ICT comes in: The easiest way to 'write down' sign language is by using sign language videos. This opens new possibilities for communication.

3 Sign Language and ICT

There are several ways of using ICT in connection with sign language. First, you can use it directly for the communication or to provide the deaf with captions; second, you can use ICT to teach deaf people their (written) national language, and, third, you can teach hearing people sign language.

3.1. Communication via ICT

During the last few years, the new communications technologies have opened many possibilities for the deaf. First came the fax, which quickly became a lifeline for most deaf people, allowing them to communicate with hearing people. The text telephone or TTY [2] might have been even better, because it allows for real-time communication, but only few hearing people had such a device. This was followed by the Short Message Service (SMS) which allowed them to communicate quickly and easily with each other - in spite of limitations like the 160 character-limit. Sometimes the unreliability of this service were messages might get lost or arrive days or weeks later. Many of the deaf especially the younger generation keep their communicator or their mobile phone close at hand to check for incoming messages. Chat is used in various forms by both hearing and deaf people.

[1] For a brief description and comparison of these systems (with examples), cf. [8].

[2] For a discussion of text telephones, cf. [9].

Although SMS is still in widespread use, nowadays mobile phones allow even for real-time video communication. In Austria, one company which specializes in video mobile phones even gave two such phones to each provincial Deaf association so that they could try it out, and there are special offers for deaf people. Another much cheaper alternative is to record what you are signing and send this file to the other person as a video-mail. Video communication is also possible by rather expensive videophones and the PC. There is no shortage of video conference programs widely available. For example, the MSN Messenger. Most of these target companies, where hearing employees want to see the other person's face while talking to them. Therefore not all of these programs are suitable for sign language communication usually because of the small size of the picture. This shows only the face instead of the whole upper body. The video quality is not good enough to allow for fluid motions and the signing is difficult to understand.

Some of these programs, however, were developed in conjunction with deaf people: e.g. "TeleSIP" by Siemens Switzerland, "Allan ec" by the Swedish company Omnitor, and "MMX" by the Swedish company Netwise (formerly Envilogg) [3]: They permit for sign language communication as long as the connection is good enough and a high speed connection is vital (i.e. broadband).

Video telephony which may be defined as "remote communication via terminals, capable of transmitting moving pictures between a sender and a receiver reciprocally" [11] is of special value to the deaf, other groups can profit from this mode of communication as well:

> There are many applications of video communication for disabled people. Perhaps the most obvious is the possibility that it offers to people who are pre-lingually deaf and use Sign Language as their preferred mode of communication. Another application is for people who are hard of hearing and will benefit greatly if they can have a voice telephone conversation accompanied by an image of the person they are speaking to. They get support from lip reading and facial expressions. Still another category is persons who have cognitive problems, such as those with intellectual disabilities or those who suffer from dementia. More applications, are as support for elderly and home bound people whose quality of life has been shown to improve when they get access to video telephony. Perhaps it applies still more in cases of emergency. Indeed, there are also applications for people who are visually impaired. In these cases the transmission can be used as a "remote eye" or, in case of partial sight, as an enhancing medium in remote education [11].

3.1.1 Relay Centers

In contrast to other countries such as Switzerland or the USA, only a few authorities in Austria such as the Social Welfare Office were provided with TTYs in Austria. This device has mostly gone out of use, even with the deaf, replaced by fax, e-mail and SMS. While those forms of written communication have their uses, hearing

[3] For a discussion of the various programs and their advantages and disadvantages, see [10].

people prefer the phone for quick and easy communication. Although deaf people are often busy sending SMS to each other or even to hearing friends or colleagues, no real-time communication is possible. Unless the other person answers, it is not even known whether the message has arrived and was understood. Even if it has, who else might have seen it apart from the intended recipient. The Austrian deaf do not like to write to hearing people especially those they do not know well, because they know that they will usually make some spelling and grammar mistakes.

Moreover, even if you know or can obtain the e-mail address, fax or SMS number of an authority or company, there is no guarantee that a hearing person will bother to answer such a message, especially if an ongoing communication is necessary. Imagine, for instance, asking for information from the tax office via SMS, or making an appointment at the doctor's where usually several questions require answers. There are even some cases where a failure to communicate may have dangerous consequences. For example, when a deaf person becomes sick and sends a fax to the doctor, patiently waiting for the answer, while there is only a tape running that the doctor is on holiday. If you do get an answer, the information will usually be condensed, or you will get only partial information, because the hearing party may not write adequate answers. This is especially so when several messages must be interchanged

A solution to this problem was found more than a decade ago. This was the introduction of so-called relay centers, which help to send messages between deaf and hearing people. In the older, text-based version, the deaf person contacted the relay center (usually via TTY) and wrote their part of the conversation. The Communications Assistant (CA) in the relay center then phoned the respective hearing party and relayed the message. The spoken answer of the hearing person was written down by the CA and sent back to the deaf person, thus allowing for real-time communication and instant feedback. The same is of course possible in the other direction. That is the call can be initiated by a hearing person. This allows the authorities as well as companies to actively contact deaf people.

With the advance in video and telecommunications technology, writing is no longer necessary as the relay center can be contacted via PC or videophone, and the deaf person can simply sign whatever they want to say. The signed message is then translated by an interpreter in the relay center. It then phones the hearing party and vice versa.

For the hard-of-hearing, unassisted phone communication may be possible, depending on their hearing loss. However, with unknown people or if there is any noise in the background, it soon comes down to guesswork. In this case, a relay center can help. While the hard-of-hearing usually have no difficulty reading and writing and thus can easily use text relay, video communication offers the advantage of additional lip-reading (also without involving a relay center). It is also possible to speak and get only the answer in written form (Voice Carry-Over or VCO).

A US-company has also found a way to improve phone conversations with a special device called the CapTel phone[4]. It is equipped with a display, which is connected to a text relay. The CA listens to the conversation and repeats everything the hearing participant says, which is then automatically written down by a speech-

[4] http://www.captionedtelephone.com/index.phtml

recognition software. This software has to be specially 'trained' to the user's voice and therefore the CA is necessary as a go-between. The text appears on the display, and if any clarification is needed, the hard-of-hearing user can listen to the answer and read it simultaneously.

Speech-impaired users will also profit from such a relay center. Most of them will probably want to use Hearing Carry-Over (HCO), where the speech-impaired user writes their part of the conversation and listens to the answer themselves. There also exists a special service called 'speech-to-speech relay', where specially trained CAs listen to the speech-impaired user and repeat whatever they say to the conversation partner.

Naturally, the communications assistants and interpreters working at the relay center are well-trained and obliged to keep every conversation completely confidential.

3.1.1.1. Relay Center Austria

While relay centers like those described above are commonplace in the USA, Switzerland, Sweden and other European countries, the technology and the range of services greatly differ. For an overview, cf. [10] and [12]. An Austrian relay center as yet does not exist. Dating back to an EU-workshop hosted by the Center for Sign Language and Deaf Communication (Zentrum fuer Gebaerdensprache und Hoerbehindertenkommunikation, ZGH) at the University of Klagenfurt in 2000 (Final report [13]) The ZGH tried to implement such a relay center in Austria.

In 2004, the Carinthian Social Welfare Office agreed to fund a six-month 'preparatory project' to provide the basis for a "Relay Center Austria" (RCA). Collaborators in the ZGH will evaluate existing relay centers and prepare a 'best practice' strategy on how to best implement such a center. Text and video relay centers in Switzerland, Sweden and the USA were also visited and there was also an Internet search which led to many e-mail contacts with people and companies involved in the relay business. As it turned out, the delay worked to our advantage, as most relay centers had to include older devices such as older brands of videophones which offered either text relay or video relay. Usually, the text relays came first, and when video was available, new companies providing this service were developed. Ideally, the relay center uses multimedia software integrating video, text and voice, so that each user can choose whatever combination works best for them. Various programs were evaluated for our purposes. For sign language, at least 15-20 frames per second are needed, and the delay must be as small as possible, in order to guarantee fluent communication.

A lot of work went into establishing a legal basis for a relay center, which is essential for its continued existence because of the guaranteed long-term funding. Mostly, this legal basis concerns either some kind of anti-discrimination law such as the Americans with Disabilities Act in the USA or equal access to telecommunications in Switzerland and Germany. Following the Swiss and German examples, we had a first look at the Austrian telecommunications law, which is vague on this subject. The first talks with telecommunications companies showed that the funding of a pilot relay center on a voluntary basis as is currently the case in Germany is not a very likely option. In Germany the Deutsche Telekom agreed to fund a three-year project.

The Austrian Sign Language (Oesterreichische Gebaerdensprache, OEGS) has finally been recognized by the Austrian parliament in an amendment to the Austrian constitution. Services for people with special needs not explicitely stated will have to be negotiated with the government individually. If the result is not satisfactory, a recently founded association which can institute proceedings against discriminating regulations, the so-called 'Klagsverband' can get involved. Both parties are obliged to undergo mediation first and if they cannot agree on an acceptable solution, the case can then be taken to court, a practice which is new for Austria.

What makes the RCA different from other relay centers is that our express aim is that the users should be able to contact it with any user end-device. There have been earlier attempts at implementing a relay center, where the users had to buy a special brand of videophone. Ideally both with stationary and mobile devices, and that the service is not limited to relay. The RCA is meant to be a kind of encompassing service center for the deaf, the hearing- and the speech-impaired.

As a first step, the core service or the relay center will be implemented, providing its users with multimedia communication. That is, integrating video, text and voice. However the service is funded, users should not be obliged to pay more for their call than a hearing user would pay for the same telephone call. The service itself is free and only the phone call to the hearing user must be paid.

The relay center allows also 'Remote Interpreting': The hearing and deaf parties are both in the same room, while the interpreter is present only via video. This saves the interpreters a lot of time and expense; for example, they will no longer have to drive for two hours to interpret for half an hour. Naturally, not all situations are suitable for Remote Interpreting such as in a court or in the hospital where a 'live' interpreter is preferable. For short questions, discussions at work and such, this is a way to battle the acute lack of interpreters in Austria. If this is possible with a video mobile phone, you practically have an 'interpreter in your pocket'.

An additional automatic conversion allows to change the format of a text into another format, that is, a TTY message into a fax message or an e-mail. Although this is not a vital service, it may sometimes facilitate communication as hearing and deaf people may use different technologies. For example, only a few hearing people have a TTY, and not all of them have a fax machine.

The RCA should also order the interpreter. Basically, what you do when you need an interpreter in most of the Austrian provinces is to acquire a list of the phone numbers of the official Austrian sign language interpreters. You then try to contact each of them until you find one who is willing to do the job. If you pick the wrong time or day, the chances are that nobody is available as there are very few full-time interpreters. Following the example of the Swiss relay center PROCOM, people should simply contact the RCA and tell them when and where they need an interpreter. One way of keeping track of the interpreters could be a database where each interpreter fills in the times they are available and special preferences. The details of cooperation have still to be arranged with the Association of the Austrian Sign Language Interpreters (Oesterreichischer Gebaerdensprach-DolmetscherInnen-Verband).

Very important is some kind of alert for the deaf. This includes both an official alert in case of fire, or civil defense, and a private emergency; cf. 3.3.3.

At a later date, e-learning will be included. The courses will be both aimed at deaf and hearing people, cf. 3.2. Another service that could be added at a later date is sending in difficult texts and receiving them back in either in 'easy-to-read' form or in a sign language.

There will also be news and information in sign language. There have been some attempts in Austria by the Austrian company "equalizent" with their Internet news project "SignTime". It is very difficult to find funding for a longer time. Using the relay center as an 'umbrella organization' and having both video technology and interpreters already within the center, success should be possible.

The competence center should also provide a platform for the target groups where they can organize themselves. It will contain community features such as chatrooms, schedules for different events, etc. and there will be the possibility of entering a user profile into a database so that users can find expert advice or friends with similar interests.

Such a relay center has many advantages: it helps the users to integrate with modern society, both in their professional and their private lives. They not need to depend on their friends and relatives to make their calls for them. Phone skills are also a vital part of today's business life. With remote interpreting, employers need not fear frequent communication problems.

3.1.2. Electronic alternatives

There are electronic alternatives to a relay center and human communication assistants and interpreters, although they do not work well or only in special circumstances as yet.

For years, research has been done on systems for speech recognition, speech and sign language synthesis, with varying success. Machine translations always suffer from problems. These problems are even worse, when there are important structural differences as is the case with spoken/written languages and sign language. An instance, the use of three-dimensional space.

In Austria, one of the telecommunications providers tried to offer a simple service to help the deaf communicate with hearing people via the phone, using the automatic transformation of written texts into spoken language. An SMS was read to a hearing person by an artificial voice. As such services did not work well as the messages often arrived garbled. Internationally, some relay centers offer a similar service, where the message is read by a human. Blind people could use this service in the other direction, by having text messages read to them without the need for a special reading device.

There were also efforts to use hand-held devices which could 'speak' written texts, in order to help the deaf directly communicate with the hearing. While this is a possibility, typing takes the user much longer than simply speaking or in this case signing.

A logical next step is therefore the use of avatar technology (i.e. a computer animation of a virtual human). One of the projects trying to guarantee an improved access to information, services and facilities for sign language users is ViSiCAST [5]. A practical application of such an avatar is the system TESSA (Text and Sign Support Assistant), which is intended to help with the communication with deaf customers in British post offices. The signs of the native signer are first captured as motion data via sensors affixed to the body of the signer. The post office clerks talk into a microphone, while the system generates the respective signs (currently, not all phrases can be correctly identified by the system). For details, cf. [14] and [15] [6].

There are different opinions of such systems: while some people - especially the hearing ones - regard them as rather helpful, there are also fears (especially within the deaf community) that the deaf might be forced to communicate only with electronic systems in the future. Nevertheless, if the technology can be made to work independently from context, TESSA and its successors might prove very useful.

In Sweden, the project SYNFACE was aimed at hard-of-hearing people [7]. A 'talking face', controlled by the incoming telephone speech signal should make it easier for hearing-impaired people to have phone conversations, by allowing them to lip-read simultaneously.

3. 2. Sign Language and E-Learning

3.2.1. E-Learning for the Deaf

As sign language can best be recorded in the form of a sign language video, e-learning (in the form of bilingual education) is ideal for deaf people.

In Austria courses written in German for deaf people are especially important. The ZGH has some experience in this area. We believe that it is best to use the target language, written German, as a basis, supplemented with sign language videos, should the users have problems understanding the text. The deaf can first try to read the text on their own, without additional help. If any of the words are too difficult or if the meaning is not clear, a help function explains everything in sign language, according to this principle [4].

> As deaf people cannot hear spoken languages well enough to learn in this way, they need a special form of bilingual education, where a sign language gives the linguistic and cognitive base and the written/spoken language is 'anchored' to the first system as a parallel but second language. Written language is of great importance to deaf people. Naturally, if they are to be integrated into the hearing society. They must have all written information at their disposal. The goal of offering them written language competence people with hearing comparable to people with hearing subjects can only be reached if

[5] http://www.visicast.sys.uea.ac.uk/Visicast_index.html

[6] For more publications on the subject of virtual signing, cf. the ViSiCAST publications: http://www.visicast.sys.uea.ac.uk/Public.html#Publications

[7] http://www.speech.kth.se/synface/

their instruction is improved. ICT is expected to play an important role in this task.

Some examples of our work will serve to illustrate what can be done in this area. That is, German courses and English for the deaf on the Internet.

3.2.1.1. Leonardo: Internet as a potential source of new employment possibilities for the deaf

In this part of the Leonardo da Vinci Programme, several courses for the deaf were developed and held in the partner countries Czech Republic, Austria, Flemish part of Belgium and United Kingdom. These included computer skills such as Internet and web page design, the respective written national languages, computer typography and Internet-related job-seeking skills. The materials for this course include textbooks and was partially accompanied by CD-ROMs.

An added bonus was the collection of standardized signs for grammar and computer terminology. The signs were discussed during meetings of deaf people from all over the country. The signs they agreed on were then filmed and stored in the form of video clips on a CD-ROM. These signs provide a basis for future courses so as to avoid confusion because the signs from different regions are used interchangeably. Interpreters can now draw on a unified terminology.

3.2.1.2. The Course Editor

Within a project aimed at introducing a new, officially recognized training for deaf teachers of sign language, the ZGH developed a written German course for future teachers. The on-line modules of this course will allow the students to look up information about German grammar and to practice it by doing exercises on their own.

For this multimedia course, we teamed up with the Austrian Research Center Seibersdorf to develop an electronic tool called "Course Editor". With this tool, exercises for courses can be created. The design of the so-called masks or templates for the exercises can be individually changed, according to the designer's wishes. The pool of finished exercises, courses may be copied and used as basis for new courses. These in turn can be added to the pool. Possible exercise types include multiple choice, close tests, complementing or merging sentences, matching text and pictures. There are currently 15 masks.

For sign language courses and language courses intended to show the contrast between spoken/written languages and sign language, exercises using videos which matching signed sentences with their translations need to be defined as a new project.

Although the course editor was originally intended for a German course, it is not limited to a single language. The course editor can be adapted to whatever exercises and videos the designer chooses. Different languages, are included by swapping the contents. The exercises can be tailored by the instructor according to the needs of the respective group of students.

In the German course, the students can do the exercises in whatever order they like; as there is no fixed course structure. The user simply chooses a subject of interest to them, for example The Present Tense, and can then read the respective grammar explanations or watch the accompanying videos in Austrian Sign Language the student may then do the various exercises. These are taken from an exercise pool, using a random generator, so that the students will get new exercises each time they access the course.

There are three levels of complexity: beginners, intermediate and advanced. Normally, the program will show all three levels one after the other for each exercise type, but the students may skip any if they do not want to do them or do not feel competent enough.

For the easier levels, feedback is sometimes inherent; for example, with drag-and-drop exercises, wrong choices will not stay in place. There is also a special button which allows the students to call up the correct solution and with another click on this button, they can repeat the exercise. In the cases where the feedback is explicit, this takes the form of red (wrong) and green (correct) boxes around the respective word, phrase, etc. It may take the form of a green hook and a red 'X' (see Fig. 1). In this way, mistakes are made visible unobtrusively. There are no grades, so that the deaf students are not feeling as if they were back at school again. This feature was included as an express wish of the deaf participants.

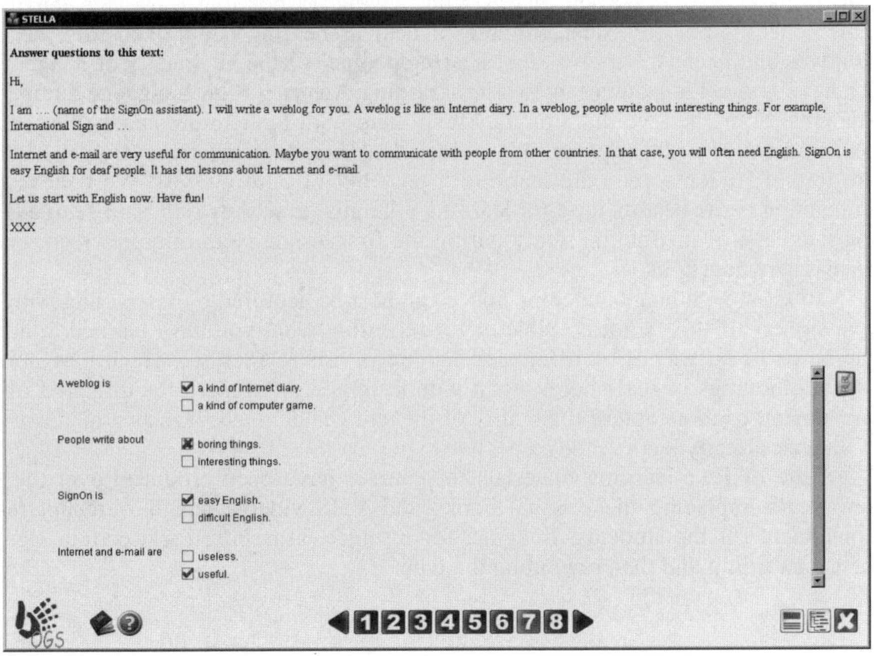

Fig. 1. An example for an exercise (answer questions) developed with the course editor

3.2.1.3. Sign On

The EU-project "Sign On - English for Deaf Sign Language Users on the Internet" [8] is a cooperative project between Austria, Finland, Iceland, the Netherlands, Norway, Spain, and the United Kingdom (October 2004 - September 2007). It is aimed at deaf people who use a sign language as their first or preferred language and are not complete beginners. That is, they are e-mail and Internet literate and have a basic competence of English.

The goals of the project are to teach deaf people some skills, strategies and to give them the confidence they need to exchange e-mails in written English and to read information on English language website. One of the target groups are deaf researchers attending international conferences and wanting to stay in contact with people from other countries afterwards. Sign bilingual learning materials (ten lessons in written English, national sign languages and International Sign) will be produced and intended both for individual study and the classroom.

The outcomes/products will include a bilingual phrase book, a website and a mailing list for students to practice their skills in a realistic context situation.

3.2.2. Learning Sign Language

For the deaf, it is important that as many people as possible learn sign language. This concerns not only deaf children of deaf or hearing people and their hearing relatives and friends, but also other hearing people. At the University of Klagenfurt, we have noticed a growing interest for learning Austrian Sign Language among the students. Some believe that this may help them with their future career. For example, students of pedagogy, and others have deaf friends or relatives. However, there are lots of students, who are learning it only out of pure interest. We believe that immersion is the best method for learning a language, so Austrian Sign Language is the language of instruction. Only during the first lesson is an interpreter present to answer any questions.

Naturally, sign language competence can best be acquired by interacting with native signers. If this is not possible or for repeating what you have learned at home, the second-best way is by using sign language videos. Pictures which may consist of line-drawings or real photos, even with little arrows to mark the direction of the movement, cannot capture the reality of the sign. They may serve as a memory-aid, if one has already learned the respective sign.

At the ZGH, e-learning materials for courses have been produced over the last few years, replacing the original books and VHS videos, which were not really convenient for the students. Imagine, for instance, searching for a certain sign by first forwarding and then rewinding the tape.

[8] The website of the project can be accessed at www.signon.fi.

3.2.2.1. Austrian Sign Language Course "OEGS 1" on CD-ROM

Although the students in our sign language courses are very motivated, they had difficulty remembering the signs and the grammar over a longer period of time and they kept asking us for a study tool. To fulfill this request, we developed a course on CD-ROM with a local software firm.

The first six lessons of the original course used at the university were adapted for a multimedia course. The next six lessons are to follow in a new project). The exercises remained mostly the same, while the PC took over the part of the teacher. True to our philosophy, only native signers appear in the videos. Mostly, sign language is used for example for the feedback. Only the instructions and grammar explanations are in written German, but this will also change in the second part of the CD-ROM.

The six lessons have all the same structure: Dialogs illustrating the main topic of the lesson. That is, description of people, are followed by exercises (an example is given in Fig. 2) and for games. The main grammar points are explained together with videos of sample sentences. Notes on deaf culture are intended to prevent hearing people from making common faux-pas. That is politely walking around two deaf people instead of crossing between them. Individual signs can be looked up at the end of each lesson or in an overall alphabetical list. For details of the contents, see [16].

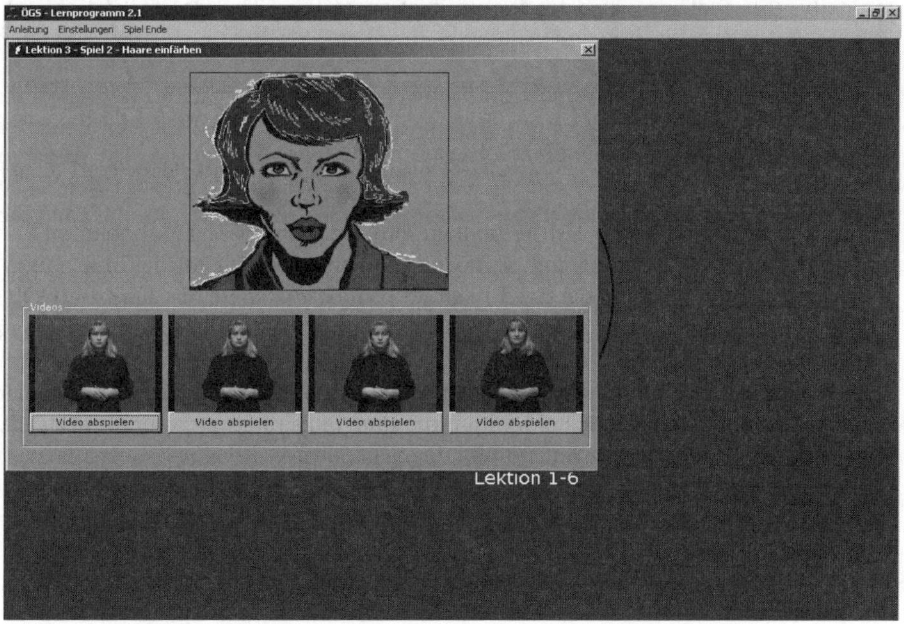

Fig. 2. Exercise for practicing the signs for the different colors

The exercises and games often take the form of drag-and-drop or matching videos and pictures/translations. Most of the exercises use a random number generator. The pictures for example are either completely different or at least they will appear in different order. That is that the students cannot simply memorize the correct solution.

Feedback is sometimes automatic with drag-and-drop, where wrong choices revert to their original place and are sometimes signed the videos are chosen by a random generator to avoid boredom. There is no rigid structure to the course: although complete beginners would be wise to do the lessons in the correct order. They can also choose to pick out the parts that interest them most.

The course is not intended as a stand-alone product, although it can be used as such. We recommend it is desirable to attend a course so as to meet and have fave to face contact with deaf people.

The reaction to the CD-ROM was very positive, and it won the "Europaeisches Sprachensiegel 2004" (European Language Quality Seal) prize. As it was programmed without static parameters, its framework could be used for other sign languages or spoken languages by changing the videos and some of the data.

3.2.2.2. The Lesson Manager

Originally, this tool was used for the production of the CD-ROM "OEGS 1" (cf. 3.2.2.1.), but it can be used independently. It allows the linking of sign language videos, glosses and written text.

Imagine, for instance, that you want to link a signed dialog with its translation. After loading a video file into the program, it can be split manually into smaller parts, such as phrases or sentences. Normal control elements are used. The user can work either at normal speed or choose to view the file frame by frame. Each of the pieces can then be linked to the name of the signer, the respective gloss(es) and the translation (see Fig. 3).

A preview function allows the user to check that the linking is correct. If not, changes are possible. The latest version of the Lesson Manager allows not only the exchange of glosses and text, but also the re-assigning of beginning and end points of the video.

The program is in German and English; but it can easily be adapted for other languages using a built-in function which requires only the translation of the German/English terms into the new language.

3.2.2.3. Sign-IT and the Klagenfurt database of signs

Sign-IT[9] was a two-year project funded by the Austrian Federal Ministry for Education, Science and Culture. It was done by the Center for Sign Language in cooperation with the University of Graz (sign language interpreter training) and the higher education institution "Joanneum", also located in Graz.

---

[9] The website of the project can be accessed at www.sign-it.at. The database can be found under the heading 'ÖGS-Lexikon'.

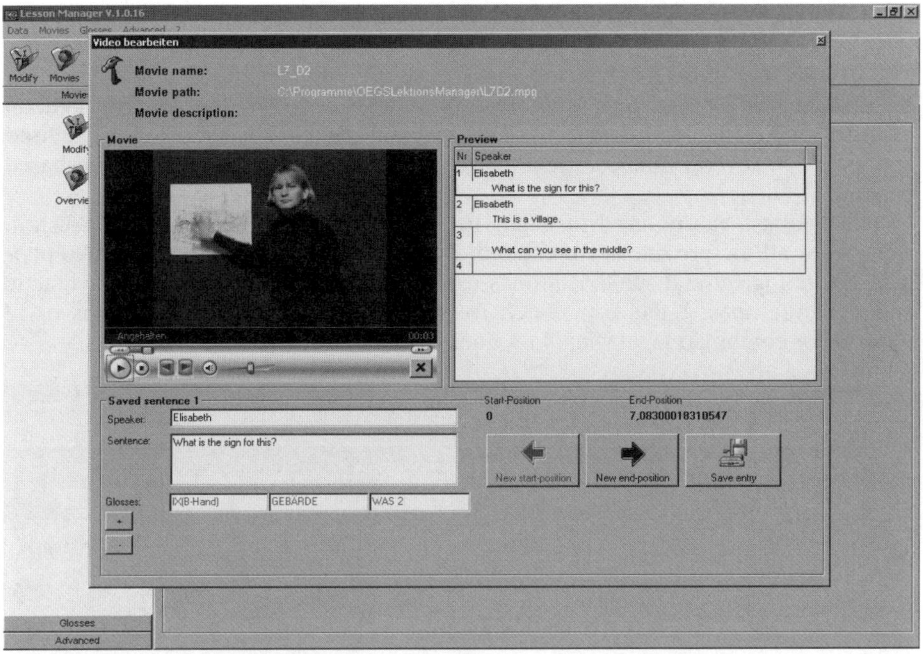

Fig. 3. Working screen of the Lesson Manager

Because sign language is taught in Austria only at two universities (Graz and Klagenfurt), not all the people interested in learning it can attend the lecture courses. The aim of the project was to develop e-learning for students of Austrian Sign Language so that they could also learn it individually. By making OEGS available to any interested person, the project would also serve to raise awareness of sign language as a minority language.

The e-learning part is still only a pilot and consists of an on-line e-learning platform which contains courses on deaf history, deaf culture and it allows communication between teachers and students. A CD-ROM for individual study is available. That is mainly aimed at interpreters and contain structured lessons, exercises and vocabulary together with an on-line database.

The database was originally developed by the Center for Sign Language (cf. 3.2.2.3.1.) and modified for this project. Signs from the different provinces of Austria were collected during meetings of deaf people and the videos then entered into the database. This lexicon not allows interested people to look up regional variants and even to start individual list of signs. Over time it may also lead to a 'soft' standardization of OEGS.

3.2.2.3.1. The Klagenfurt database for sign language lexicons

The first version of the database was developed for a project aimed at implementing a special server for deaf people in 1997/98. It was funded by the Austrian Federal Ministry of Science and Transport. This original database has since been revised and extended several times; currently, we are working on a completely web-based version.

The database can be used for signs from different sign languages. For Austria, signs from all the provinces are entered. Not only formational properties like phonetic-phonological and sublexical ones can be described, but also morphosyntactic and semantic ones. Users can search for single entries, properties of signs or in isolation or combination, cf. Fig. 4 or via semantic fields.

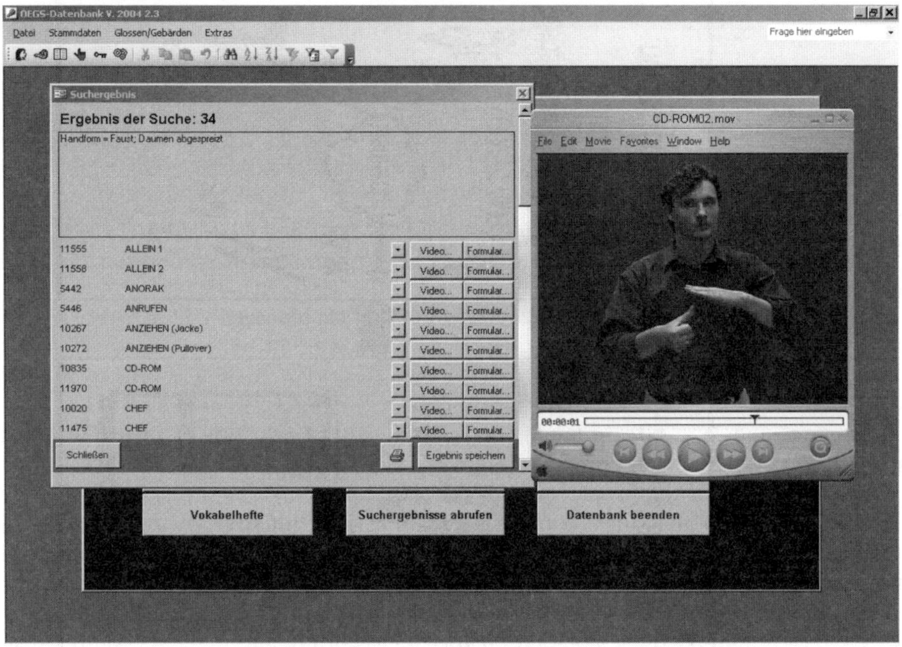

Fig. 4. Example for a search for signs with a special handshape

The software is based on the programs Oracle, Access, Java and HTML. As for the linguistic concept, we used a blend of Liddell & Johnson's [17] Movement-and-Hold model, a modified HamNoSys [6] and the SignPhon category system [18]. The main characteristics are the iconic arrangement of sign components and the open sets of categories/parameters and category values. New categories and values can be added at any time, if necessary. For details, see [19].

3.3. Barrier-free Access to Information for Deaf People

Nowadays, one of the keywords of our modern society is 'barrier-free access'. Ramps have to be built for wheelchair users, websites have to be modified so that vision-impaired people will be able to read them, to name just a few of the measures taken to realize this goal. Although all of these are necessary, deaf people are mostly left out, especially where access to information is concerned. One way to overcome obstacles such as a lack of foreign language knowledge as much information is in English only and poor reading skills is by the use of sign language videos. For discussions of the situation of deaf and hearing-impaired people with respect to the Internet, see [20] and [21].

3.3.1. Barrier-free access to the Internet

One of the requirements of our communication society is access to information on the Internet. A lot has already been done for barrier-free access, but sign language is usually seen as only a desirable addition, not a top priority.

Take, for instance, the Web Content Accessibility Guidelines (WCAG) of the Web Accessibility Initiative (WAI) [10], where sign language is mentioned as a 'non-text equivalent of text'. The focus is still on 'clear and simple' written language, which also benefits sign language users. While this is true, sign language would be preferred by most deaf people. The lack of sign language videos may be due to simple thoughtlessness. Hearing people without direct contact to the deaf community are usually convinced that deaf people can easily compensate by reading written texts. The costs of preparing such videos may act as a deterrent.

For example, in an Austrian integrative project producing a barrier-free version of the European Computer Driving License (ECDL) for people with special needs, easy written language was used for hearing-impaired people [22]. The project was intended to supply deaf users with additional sign language videos. Once again, the costs were so high that sign language was relegated to a later stage and the deaf will in the meantime have to make do with the written version only.

There are some initiatives by European governments to mend matters. In 2004, the German Federal Ministry of Health and Social Security included in some of its web pages additional sign language videos [11]. They received enthusiastic feedback, but an accompanying survey indicated that the users would like more such videos. From all the people interviewed, only 10 % understood the contents in written form and, more than 89 % needed sign language to really understand the texts [23].

A similar venture has been started in Austria in spring 2005. There is a special website managed by the Austrian authorities which deals with e-government [12]. Citizens can get information from the various ministries, print out forms, etc. The project itself consists of two phases: In the first phase, the necessary signs were

---

[10] Cf. http://www.w3.org/WAI/intro/wcag.php.

[11] Cf. http://www.bmgs.bund.de/deu/gra/gehoer/ghv_start.cfm.

[12] Cf. www.help.gv.at.

agreed upon during a deaf conference and filmed. In the second phase, information texts will also be signed.

There are also some websites - mostly maintained by deaf associations or institutions/organizations which work with the deaf and use sign language videos. An excellent example of a bilingual website is Sign Community of the British Deaf Association [13], where users are free to choose between British Sign Language and a text version.

As for news and information, a European example of good practice is the Swiss "Focus-5 TV" [14], which is run by deaf people and covers many subjects, ranging from the Deaflympics to films for children. This excellent website can really be compared to "TV for deaf people". In Austria, the “Oesterreichischer Gehoerlosenbund” [15] (Austrian Deaf Association) offers news in the form of video clips in Austrian Sign Language and text on their website. Since January 2005, they also cooperate with BIZEPS, which is an association which offers advice to people with special needs and their relatives, publishes chosen bilingual news on their website “BIZEPS-INFO” [16] .

Unfortunately, such websites are few and far between. Although video technology has come a long way, producing sign language videos is still a time-consuming and expensive process. Until there are new technological developments, sign language will probably remain limited to those websites which take a special interest in the deaf community and maybe a few official websites.

One solution might be that demonstrated by the EU-project eSign a further development of ViSiCAST, which aims to provide sign language on websites, using avatar technology. It is currently working on local Government websites in Germany, the Netherlands and the United Kingdom. They claim that, although the technology is still in development, virtual signing can be made even better than using videos of real signers. Changing small sections of the signing can be done quickly. This is true for updates as videos can be downloaded faster and do not take up much space on Internet servers [17].

3.3.2. Captions and sign language inserts

Deaf people miss information and entertainment that hearing people take for granted.

The cheapest and easiest method to improve the situation is to use captioning [18]. In Austria, even lip-reading from the screen is usually not possible for deaf people

[13] Cf. www.signcommunity.org.uk.

[14] Cf. www.focus-5.tv.

[15] Cf. http://www.oeglb.at/.

[16] Cf. http://www.bizeps.or.at/oegs.php.

[17] For a detailed description of the project and demo video clips, cf. http://www.sign-lang.uni-hamburg.de/eSIGN/.

[18] For a brief history of closed captioning in the USA, cf. the website of the National Captioning Institute (http://www.ncicap.org/Docs/history.htm).
Similar services using teletext have been established in many other countries, e.g. in New Zealand (cf. http://www.captioningnz.co.nz/history.php).

unless they know English as most of the films have been dubbed. A solution has been found by spreading of cheap DVDs. The Austrian deaf usually wait for the DVD and then watch the film with special captions for hearing-impaired people. Most of the films in television have also been dubbed. Captions can be added, but only for a rather small percentage of the program.

Sign language inserts are possible and even better. In Austria there is only a single news program shown weekly which uses an interpreter. With the advance of digital TV, a daily news program is signed as well, but the drawback here is that one needs a special device. A positive example is the German TV station "Phoenix", which broadcasts news with sign language daily [19] .

The ZGH has also been experimenting with sign language inserts. The University of Klagenfurt has its own TV team, called "Campus-TV". They produce news items which are of interest to the staff and the students. In cooperation with Campus-TV, the ZGH has added inserts of native signers to some of these shorts.

Plays and even music are sometimes interpreted by sign language interpreters during special performances for deaf people. At international conferences, for example, sign language interpreters and stenographers providing real-time captioning by typing almost literally what is spoken are a common sight. Automatic speech recognition, which can be defined as "the independent, Computer-driven transcription of spoken language into readable text in real time" [24] is another possibility. Currently, such systems must usually be trained to recognize a speaker's individual voice characteristics in order to achieve a high degree of accuracy. Future developments may succeed in making them speaker-independent. A hand-held device which can translate everything that is said into text would be a valuable aid for deaf and hard-of hearing people. For the deaf a translation into sign language would be even better.

3.3.3. Alert/Emergency

3.3.3.1. Alert

In many countries, the public are alerted by using an acoustic signal. Sirens are used for fire alerts or in civil-defense situations. Further information, such as instructions to stay at home, keep all the windows closed is available via television, radio, or a telephone number. The same holds for traffic news: when, for instance, a person driving in the wrong direction is reported, hearing drivers will receive this announcement via their car-radios. Not being aware of such alerts or some vital piece of information can lead to life-threatening situations. Deaf people often have to rely on SMS messages from hearing friends or relatives to keep them informed. During an emergency, such services are liable to break down because the communication system overloads. A good example for this is an account by a deaf Australian on what happened during the Canberra bushfires. They could only rely on the behaviour of people on the street. They almost tired to escape on a route that was closed due to the fire [25].

---

[19] Cf. http://www.phoenix.de/startseite/1.1.htm.

Within buildings, special technical aids can help with an evacuation alert. These include devices which signal an emergency with strobe flashing lights or pager-like devices which vibrate to signal a message. One of the latter, the so-called Deaf Alerter [20] also emits a piercing audible tone which can be used by rescue personnel to locate a deaf or hard-of-hearing person if they are trapped[21].

Ideally, such an alert should be transmitted via a mobile device, such as a mobile phone, which can be worn all the time. With modern phones, the user could be located and alerted to emergencies in their direct neighborhood as well as receive further information similar to other GPS-based services. SMS warnings are also possible; although those are not fool-proof as messages can be lost. Such an aid is better than nothing.

In Germany, there is a special system called SOPHIA ("Soziale Personenbetreuung - Hilfen im Alter") [22], which started as a model project in Bamberg in 2001 and was later turned into a company. Originally intended for the elderly, SOPHIA has been further developed into "SOPHIA Silence" for hearing- or speech-impaired people. A set of sensors provides data to a central office (e.g. fire, water, smoke). The system is coupled with interactive video communication. In case of an emergency, help will be alerted.

3.3.3.2. Emergency

Deaf people also have difficulties to report an emergency. In Germany, the Deutsche Schwerhoerigenbund (Association for the Hard-of-Hearing) has prepared special emergency faxes in several languages which can be filled out in advance. The deaf person has only to check which emergency service is needed, such as police, fire brigade or ambulance [27]. Deaf or hearing-impaired people can also request the police and/or fire brigade to store their personal data in the computer so that the rescue teams will know what to expect [28].

In some countries, emergency centers can be called via TTY. In the USA all 9-1-1 centers are required by The Americans with Disabilities Act (ADA) to have such a device. Some relay services also provide special emergency services. For example, the "106 Text Emergency Relay Service" of the Australian Communication Exchange (ACE) [29].

In Sweden, there is a project run by the National Post & Telecom Agency ("Post & Telestyrelsen") and the national 'Emergency Center' "SOS Alarm", where hearing- or speech-impaired people can contact the emergency center via SMS. First tests have shown that SMS messages are not always reliable as they may arrive late or not at all. In this case some kind of feedback message is essential. Further negative impressions were the lack of direct contact and the relatively long time it took to compose a message [30].

---

[20] Cf. http://www.deaf-alerter.com/website.htm.

[21] This was, for example, a problem for deaf people during World War II: not only could they not hear the sirens warning of air raids, but if they were buried alive under a collapsed house, the rescue teams would often shout for survivors and move on if they did not receive any answer [26].

[22] Cf. http://www.senivita.de/sophia/.

The Subgroup Inclusive Communications (INCOM) of the Communications Committee (COCOM) of the European Union stated:

> However, given the increasing use of SMS by deaf persons, it is the only system currently available and needs major modification and movement to other, real-time interactive systems to be suitable for an emergency situation.
>
> SMS was not designed to be used for emergency communications but as a commercial messaging service with all the inherent attributes. There needs to be more study of the use of SMS for emergency communications about its practicality both from a user and emergency services side [31].

For those deaf or hearing-impaired people whose first language is a sign language, video communication would be ideal. For example by means of a video relay center. This is not always possible yet. It is certainly an option for the future, at least until a better solution can be found. In the USA emergency calls cannot always be routed automatically to the nearest public safety answering point due to current limitations of the video relay service. It is recommended that customers use the traditional TTY relay service to avoid possible life-threatening delay [23] .

In the Final Report of the INCOM Subgroup, it is suggested among other things that to overcome these restraints,

> - it is desirable that persons with disabilities are able to call the emergency services free of charge using their ordinary communication equipment, by using the single European emergency call number '112'; the call may be handled in text or voice or video or a combination of these media [31].

4. Conclusion

While ICT has certainly done much to make deaf people's lives easier with regard to communication and information access, much remains to be done.

For example, there still remains the problem of high costs. While sign language is essential for deaf people, as long as text-to-sign, avatars, and similar solutions are still in their infancy, sign language videos will have to be produced by filming real signers. Because these videos cannot be done automatically - at least for the near future - they are not cheap. In turn, this will deter the hearing from adding them to websites, television programs, etc.

Although with the advent of the cochlear implant and genetic engineering it sometimes appeared that a universal cure for deafness was a possibility. The need for sign language and new technologies is still strong. With a world population of about 6,000 million people, there are at least 6 million deaf people worldwide for whom adequate ways of inclusion must be found. During the next decades, ICT (and especially multimedia technology) will play an important role in this regard. A

[23] Cf. e.g. the recommendation by Hands On Video Relay Services in their Frequently Asked Questions: https://secure.hovrs.com/faq/.

huge problem is in the developing countries. Although ICT could be used to improve the lot of deaf people there, obstacles are posed simply by the lack of technological access. Whatever will be done in the future, any measures should be taken in close cooperation with the deaf group itself and based on their individual needs and wishes.

5 References

The websites cited in this article are dating back to July 4, 2005.

1. Communications Committee: Access to ICT by people with disabilities and European legislation (COCOM 03-07, Working Document). European Commission Directorate-General Information Society (2003), p. 2
   http://forum.europa.eu.int/irc/DownLoad/kVe_A4JDmRGRUS7cuqGQKvSlov32p43tkeAJmGpgO1-4T5Uc-5pHofd2iCrGc-Sl/COCOM03-07.pdf
2. Boyes Braem, P.: Einfuehrung in die Gebaerdensprache und ihre Erforschung. Internationale Arbeiten zur Gebaerdensprache und Kommunikation Gehoerloser, Vol. 11 (3rd rev. ed.). Signum: Hamburg (1995)
3. Supalla, T.: The classifier system in American Sign Language. In: Craig, C. (ed.): Noun classes and categorization. Typological Studies in Language, Vol. 7. Benjamins: Amsterdam (1986) 181-214
4. Dotter, F.: Users, ICT and Politics: The Case of the Inclusion of Sign Language Communities. In: Carrasquero, J.V., Welsch, F., Oropeza, A., Mitchell, C., Välimäki, M. (eds.): Proceedings Pista 2004. International Conference on Politics and Information Systems: Technologies and Applications. Vol. 1: Informatics and Society. International Institute of Informatics and Systemics: Orlando (2004) 206-211, p. 206
5. Stokoe, W.C., Casterline, D. C., Croneberg, C.G. (eds.): A dictionary of American Sign Language on linguistic principles. New ed. Linstok: Silver Spring, MD (1976)
6. Prillwitz, S., Leven, R., Zienert, H., Hanke, T., Henning, J.: HamNoSys. Version 2.0; Hamburg Notation System for Sign Languages. An introductory guide. International Studies on Sign Language and Communication of the Deaf, Vol. 5. Signum: Hamburg (1989)
   http://www.sign-lang.uni-hamburg.de/Projects/HamNoSys.html
7. http://www.signwriting.org
8. http://www.signwriting.org/forums/linguistics/linguistics.html
9. Nordic Forum for Telecommunication and Disability: Nordic Guide to Text Telephony. NFTH 2 (2002)
   http://www.nsh.se/NFTH-Text_Telephony.pdf
10. Hilzensauer, M., Dotter, F., Maitz, M., Fruehstueck, M., Hopfgartner, A., Oberauer, J., Valentin A.-M.: Relay Center Austria: Bericht zur Projektvorbereitungsphase. Project funded by: Social Welfare Office. Zentrum fuer Gebaerdensprache und Hoerbehindertenkommunikation: Ms. Klagenfurt (2005)
11. Brodin, J., Hellström, G., Lindström, J.-I., Martin, M., Pereira, L.M., Roe, P.: New Ways of Using Video Telephony. COST 219bis Guidebook (1999), p. 4f.
    http://www.stakes.fi/cost219/videotelephony.htm
12. Roe, P R.W. (ed.): Bridging the Gap? Access to telecommunications for all people. COST 219 European Commission (2001)
    http://www.tiresias.org/phoneability/bridging_the_gap/

13. Research Center for Sign Language and Communication of the Hearing-Impaired: Preparing a European Deaf Network for Information and Communication. Project funded by: European Commission, Directorate General "Information Society" according to the Grant Agreement signed on December 30, 1999 within the framework of the program PROMISE and the Austrian Government, Ministry for Education, Science and Culture. Klagenfurt (2000)
http://www.uni-klu.ac.at/zgh/eu_projekte/2000/
14. Bangham, J.A., Cox, S.J., Elliott, R., Glauert, J.R.W., Marshall, I., Rankov, S., Wells, M.: Virtual Signing: Capture, Animation, Storage and Transmission - an Overview of the ViSiCAST Project. IEE Seminar on "Speech and language processing for disabled and elderly people", London, April 2000
http://www.visicast.sys.uea.ac.uk/Public.html#Publicity
15. Cox, S., Lincoln, M., Nakisa, M., Wells, M., Tutt, M., Abbott, S.: The Development And Evaluation Of A Speech To Sign Translation System To Assist Transactions. Int. Journal of Human Computer Interaction (accepted for publication in 2003/2004)
http://www.visicast.sys.uea.ac.uk/Public.html#Publicity
16. Hilzensauer, M.: CD-ROM on Austrian Sign Language: Course OEGS 1, Lesson 1-6. In: Miesenberger, K., Klaus, J., Zagler, W., Burger, D. (eds.): Computers Helping People with Special Needs. Proceedings from the 9th International Conference, ICCHP 2004. Paris, France, July 2004. Springer: Berlin Heidelberg (2004) 1099-1106
17. Liddell, S.K., Johnson, R.E.: American Sign Language: The phonological base. Sign Language Studies, Vol. 64 (1989) 195-277
18. Blees, M., Crasborn, O., van der Hulst, H., van der Kooij, E.: SignPhon. A database tool for phonological analysis of sign languages. Ms. Leiden (1996)
19. Krammer, K., Bergmeister, E., Dotter, F., Hilzensauer, M., Okorn, I., Orter, R., Skant, A.: The Klagenfurt database for sign language lexicons. Sign Language & Linguistics, Vol. 4, 1/2 (2001) 191-201
20. Albiez, M.: Moeglichkeiten und Grenzen der Internetnutzung fuer hoergeschaedigte Menschen. Unter Einbezug einer Praxisstudie. Schriftliche Hausarbeit zur Ersten Staatspruefung fuer das Lehramt an Sonderschulen. Universitaet Muenchen (2000)
http://www.taubenschlag.de/lernen/wissenschaft/albiez/albiez.pdf
21. Klotz, S.: Vergessene Zielgruppe des Internets? Gehoerlose und Internet - Analyse der Beduerfnisse einer Zielgruppe und Schlussfolgerungen am Beispiel Berlins. Potsdam (1998)
http://www.taubenschlag.de/klotz/arbeit.pdf
22. Integrationsprojekt "ECDL barrierefrei". Zugang zum Europaeischen Computer Fuehrerschein fuer Menschen mit Behinderungen. bit media (no year)
http://www.bitmedia.cc/images/Infopaket_ECDL_barrierefrei.pdf
23. Gebaerdensprach-Filme im Internet. Eine Umfrage vom BMGS und Gebaerdenwerk im Zeitraum vom 15. Januar - 20. Februar 2004
http://www.bmgs.bund.de/downloads/UmfrageGebaerdenvideos.pdf
24. Stuckless, R.: Developments in real-time speech-to-text communication for people with impaired hearing. In: Ross, M. (ed.): Communication access for people with hearing loss. York Press: Baltimore, MD (1994) 197-226
http://netac.rit.edu/publication/asr.html
25. Jolley, W.: When the Tide Comes In: Towards Accessible Telecommunications for People with Disabilities in Australia: A discussion paper commissioned by the Human Rights and Equal Opportunities Commission (2003), p. 82
http://www.hreoc.gov.au/disability_rights/communications/tide.htm
26. Pullen, G., Sutton-Spence, R.: Die britische Gehoerlosengemeinschaft waehrend des Zweiten Weltkriegs. In: Fischer, R., Lane, H. (eds.): Blick zurueck: Ein Reader zur Geschichte von Gehoerlosengemeinschaften und ihren Gebaerdensprachen.

Internationale Arbeiten zur Gebaerdensprache und Kommunikation Gehoerloser, Vol. 24. Signum: Hamburg (1993) 203-210

27. Deutscher Schwerhoerigenbund: Vordruck-Download-Center (no year) http://www.schwerhoerigen-netz.de/DSB/SERVICE/NOTRUFE/
28. Deutscher Schwerhoerigenbund: Befreiungs-Erklaerung fuer Menschen mit einer Behinderung zu persoenlichen Notfall-Daten (no year) http://www.schwerhoerigen-netz.de/DSB/SERVICE/NOTRUFE/VORLAGEN/befreiung.doc
29. Australian Communication Exchange: Fact Sheet Emergency Relay Service v.4.2. (no year) http://www.aceinfo.net.au/Resources/Downloads/factsheets/pdf/015ers.pdf
30. Åslund, J. Report Summary. Test of SMS - chat for emergency number 112. Netlight Consulting: Stockholm (2003) http://www.netlight.se/reports/112-SMS_Chat_Summary.pdf
31. Inclusive Communications Subgroup (INCOM) of the Communications Committee (COCOM): Report from the inclusive communications (INCOM) subgroup Draft 4.3 (INCOM 03-23, Working document 04-08). European Commission Directorate-General Information Society: Brussels (2004), p. 27 http://forum.europa.eu.int/irc/DownLoad/k4eGA8JAmjGHclh1DU-6ZFFzIXT2tTmGzX5L_0I3gjuU-SHXZ-pP74mUmAxcL1kDZzNeUsgFZ/COCOM04-08%20INCOM%20subgroup.pdf

8. Gait Training System for Computer-aided Rehabilitation

Hidetaka Ikeuchi[1], Fumitaka Kamifukumoto[2], Satoshi Arakane[3], Kengo Ohnishi[1], Keiji Imado[1], Hiroomi Miyagawa[1] And Yukio Saito[4]

[1] Oita University, Faculty of Engineering, 700 Dannoharu, Oita-Shi, 870-1192, JAPAN
{hikeuchi, ohnishi, imado, miyahiro}@cc.oita-u.ac.jp

[2] ASICS Corporation, 1-1, Minatojima-Nakamachi 7-chome, Chuo-ku, Kobe 650-8555, JAPAN

[3] Daihen Technology Institute, 1660-7 Mizoi, Kituki-shi, Oita, 873-0025 JAPAN
arakane@daihentec.co.jp

[4] Tokyo Denki University, Ishizaka, Hatoyama, Saitama 350-0311, JAPAN
saito@n.dendai.ac.jp

Abstract. This Gait Training system is designed to simulate the effects of gait training in a swimming pool. The weight of the subject is supported by a slinging system, while the subject walks on force plates placed on a round track. The slinging force is controlled by the data collected from the force plates. The purpose of the system is to control the slinging force to maintain the most effective load on the subject's lower extremity during training, and to adapt the slinging force to the subject's recovery. The training effects are evaluated on the basis of the data that are obtained from the force plate etc. This system is tested by impaired people to evaluate its performance and efficacy. A major problem of deficient body alignment of the walking posture was found as a result of the tests. We propose mounting a display so that the results of this improvement can be verified. The effects on the walking posture using the Gait Training System were also tested on normal persons. The difference of the posture in normal gait and device-supported gait is shown.

1 Introduction

Rehabilitation training is one of the fields where mechatronic and robotic systems are capable of providing effective tools for diagnosis and treatments. The process is dependent on algorithms of measurement, control, and analysis which are based on

H. Ikeuchi et al.: *Gait Training System for Computer-aided Rehabilitation*, Studies in Computational Intelligence (SCI) **19**, 207–234 (2006)
www.springerlink.com

quantitative method and data. Therefore, the operation can be made without the therapist having to work with the patient each time. The objective of this device is to develop convenient tool for the therapist to enhance treatment, but not to replace them. The device allows the treatment of multiple subjects simultaneously, or of a single subject with focus at more conditions. This provides novel alternatives in diagnosis and treatments. The device decreases the physical load in therapy treatment, both for the patient and therapist, and it modifies the cost, accuracy, repeatability, and most of all, the patient's motivation of therapeutic training. Illustrative cases in this study target gait training, conventional rehabilitation is performed using parallel bars or in a pool. Parallel bars are often used for the rehabilitation of patients with enfeebled lower limb functions while the therapist stands by the patient. The advantage is that the equipment is easy to install and to use. This training has the disadvantages in that the stability, safety, and repeatability all rely on the patient's residual ability, which can be very tense and difficult for the patient. The training in a heated swimming pool may not be so strenuous for the patient. However, the use of a pool has drawbacks due to the size and need for maintenance. Also, due to the stress on the therapist in terms of ensuring the safety of the patient in the pool.

Several gait training devices have been proposed in papers and have shown the effects of the devices in locomotor therapy. Ide et al. developed a gait training robot, AID-1 [1]. The patient walks in a circular trajectory while the arm holding the subject rotates around the center shaft. The device alleviates problems of trunk support and decreasing body weight by powering the slinging force with pneumatic control and the counter weight balancing. A load cell is installed in the arm to minimize the load variance. However, this sensor arrangement limits the measurement of the gait condition to be applied in the control. A system named Flora developed by FATEC Co. is also a sling controlled type gait assisting system which can be applied to rehabilitation [2]. This slinging controller is suspended by a metal plate in the ceiling and enables it to train the subject without the limitation of gait trajectory, although, the same limitation applies to the gait measurement technique. KineAssist [3] another drivable training and assistive device [4-6] which controls the assisting power with force sensors within the body supporting arm is able to prevent a fall, but the system requires other transducers and algorithm for fine assessments of the gait. This can be a drawback to automated rehabilitation.

Fujie et al. with Hitachi developed a power-assisted walking support device [7]. The device trains the subject to walk on an independently controllable left and right treadmill belts, while holding the body with arm rests and handles. The system is capable of providing gait training with constant speed or loading exercise mode, and also has a tripping prevention training mode. A treadmill device is a popular mechanism because of its easy-installation and ease-of-use. Though, this method lacks the sense of dynamic body movement since acceleration of the body in the direction of movement is canceled. Lokomat [8] has the same shortcoming.

In this chapter, we describe our development of a gait training system that dynamically supports the body weight with ground reaction force gained from force measuring apparatus installed on the floor. The development and control of the system is presented first. Next, the procedure and the result of using the testing device with impaired persons are described. The advantages and disadvantages of this device are determined in these tests. A field test of a mid-term training on one patient is presented. One of the issues in the practice of the system was the walking posture with the sling support. The body alignment of the subject tended to be unbalanced, that is, leaning forward or sitting in the harness. With the use of a 3-D motion capturing system, analysis of the walking posture of the impaired person is compared with the non-impaired person using the system with a normal gait. The successful outcome of installing an online camera and display for visual feed back to monitor the subject's foot location is discussed in the next section.

2 Approach

The three key features of the design of the gait training system are the dynamic and selective support, natural sense of gait, and recording of the measurement for training assessment. The first technical goal of developing our gait training system was to provide a training device that produces a similar effect as that of buoyancy in a swimming pool. Safely is provided with a support of the body weight at a tolerable level. The subject will be capable of focusing on their body movements and balance their body posture. A therapist can focus on observing and advising the subject without the worry of sustaining and propelling the subject's gait. The second goal is to implement this support so that it produces a more natural walking condition than a treadmill. We built the system so the training floor surface condition can be varied. That is to include steps or an uneven surface. Lastly, we believed it is important to dynamically control the supporting force based on the quantitative data obtained from the subject's gait. The measurement of the subject's gait must be simultaneously conducted and recorded to plan for future training conditions. The accumulation of expertise in gait analysis technique developed on the force plate system is a good way appeal to implement the system.

The experimental prototypes were developed by Saito at el. at Tokyo Denki University [9]. The system consists of 12 force plates installed in a circle, with four arms to support the subject's body weight independently while being propelled along the trajectory with the central shaft rotation motor. The force plate was designed with an aluminum honey-comb structure to be light-weight, stiff, and suitable for precise measurement of the reaction force. Also, two types of harness were designed for the subject to wear for suspension. The main feature of this system is constant dynamic adjustment of tension to support the subject. This is done by means of information obtained from ground reaction force and controlling the supporting wire tension by means of an electric motor. The load on the subject's foot on the floor is controlled within a threshold value based on the body weight set before the beginning of training. The subject senses the stimulation on the sole and other parts of the body as in a natural walk, as he is walking on the force plate, which has a solid surface. The development of the prototype, such as cumbersome hard wiring among the sensors, actuators and controller, are modified. Wireless data transferring technologies are implemented and hardware and software functions are modified for the current system developed in a joint project with Daihen Technology Institute, Oita University, and Tokyo Denki University.

3 System Configuration and Method

3.1 System Overview

Figure1 shows the concept design of the system. A slinging system supports the subject while he walks on force-measuring floor plates. The lifting power of the slinging system is constantly controlled during the training by the information obtained from the force plates. This information is forwarded to the main control unit through the high-speed digital communication system. The control signal computed in the main control unit is then sent to the slinging control unit by the communication system. Therefore, this system constantly provides the most tolerable load level to the trainee by adjusting the lifting force according to the trainee's degree of recovery. The system also provides a tool for evaluating the effect of training by displaying the training records and the force plate data.

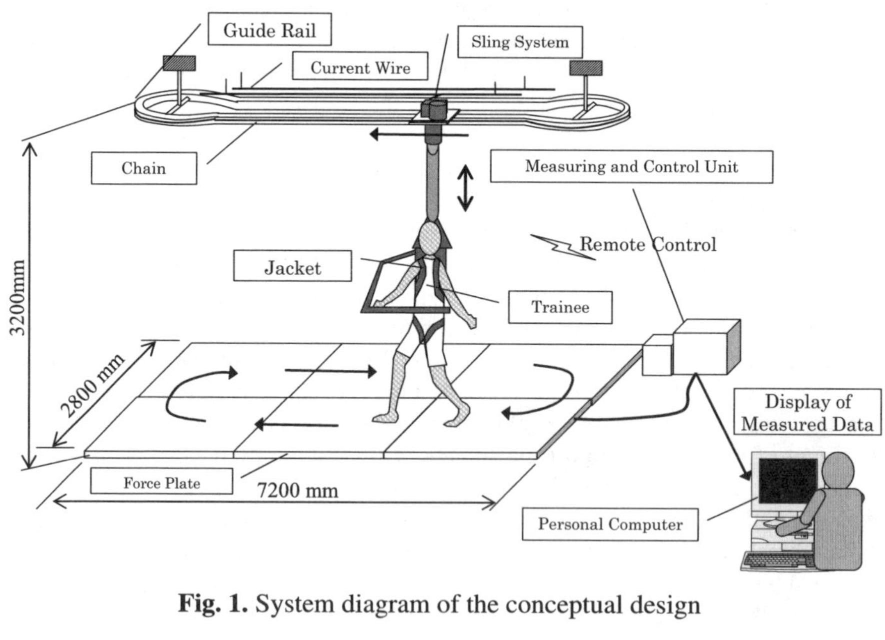

Fig. 1. System diagram of the conceptual design

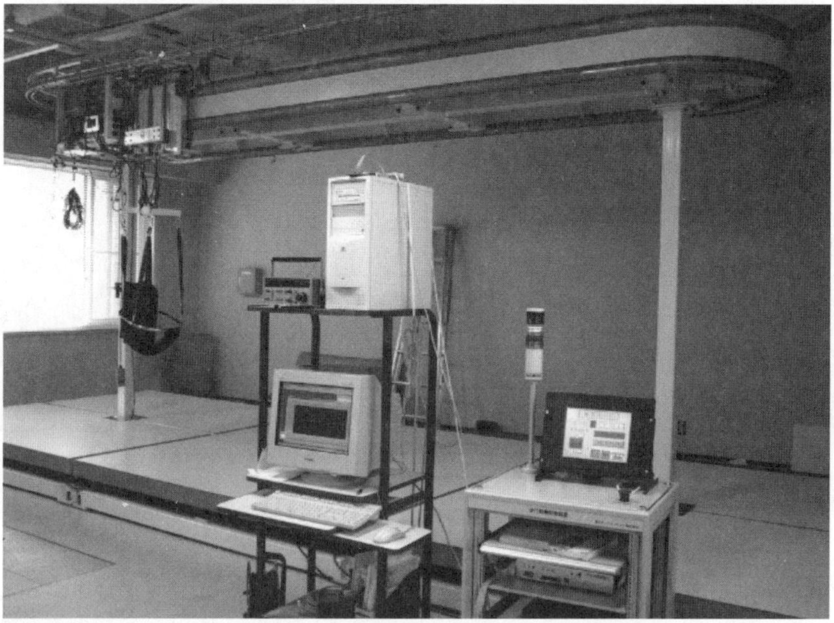

Fig. 2. Gait Training System. The right rack in the front is the main controller with a touch panel interface. The left rack is a data acquisition computer. Six force plate boards are installed for measuring the ground reaction force in gait. The sling system is mounted on a rail which circulates around the trajectory continuously. The supporting force for supporting some of the subject's body weight and the propulsive force are supplied by AC motors.

Figure 2 is the current gait training system developed. The floor area is 7.5 X 2.9 m^2, and is covered with aluminum honey-comb structured force plates. These plates have 4 force sensors at the bottom that measure the amount of pressure on them, which are applied by the subjects. The walking distance of the mean trajectory on the device is approximately 12 m. Two props support the guide rail that supports sling system. A touch panel is used for system operation. Controls for setting the load on the foot, walking speed, manual operation of the sling units, and start/stop of training are displayed.

Figure 3 shows the system diagram of the signal transmission mechanism. The sling system component supports the subject, and lifts or lowers the person according to the information from the force plates. The information for sling control is sent to the sling system component from the main control unit by Spread Spectrum Wireless Data Communications. The power for the sling system is supplied by a trolley wire; which enables the subject to walk freely without restriction.

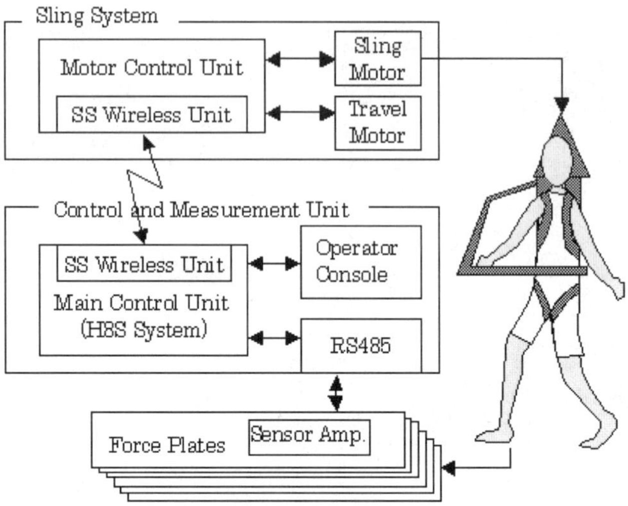

Fig. 3. System diagram of the signal transmission

3.2 Sling System Component

The sling system manages the load on the subject's foot by controlling the motor torque which produces the force on the wire to hold some of the body weight. The sling system also controls the subject's propulsion and walking speed. The traveling speed is presently set constant by the input at the touch panel. This unit is composed of a 200 W AC motor for load control, 300 W AC motor for the traveling, slinging mechanism, traveling mechanism and the computer controller. The computer has 4 functions: data reception, torque computation, traveling speed control, and slinging force control. The wire holding the trainee is connected to a ball screw nut module. Two ball spines and a ball screw shaft drive the nut vertically. The AC motor is connected to the ball screw shaft, and the generative torque is transferred to the wire through the mechanism. A brake mechanism is installed to hold the subject stationary, while a manual switch can release the brake and slowly release the subject. The switch is also used to lower the slider when transferring the patient from the wheelchair and later driving it to stand the patient upright. The range of the slider is limited so that the patient does not collapse on the floor.

3.3 Supporting Vest

To harness the subject to the sling system, supporting vests were developed. These hold and support the body weight of the patient and are connected to the slinging unit. The ease of attaching and wearing this equipment has a considerable influence on the success of the system. The training cannot be conducted repeatedly or within period of time it causes pain or complicated to fit. We tried a number of off-the-shelf products, but none of them were durable. Our supporting vests are still being further developed to meet our goal of being comfortable and allowing free movement during the gait

The equipment in Fig 4-(a) and (b) were developed with this aim. Fig.4-(a) is Type I, which was originally developed in this project. Several prototypes have been produced through trial and error to reach this design. Denim cloth is mainly used due to its flexibility and durability. The load is sustained mostly between the thighs with a soft tube, while partially supported at the trunk where the jacket is wrapped around the patients midsection. The rap-around belt type jacket provides a sense of security for maintaining body posture and is easy to wear and can be adjusted by using Velcro fastenings. A steel frame pipe holds a soft stuffed tube for the crotch in a comfortable manner. The frame is designed to hold the vertical load applied on tube while distributing the force on the body so as to not restrict the movement of the hip joint and pelvis. Many patients have remarked that this pipe works to lower the mental stress on the trainee as it can be used as a handle. The support vest is attached to the sling with 4 wires that adjust to the height of the trainee. The 4-point support of the frame pipe gives stability the body posture.

Figure 4-(b) is Type II, which utilizes a harness already on the market, a BIODEX vest, (Biodex Medical Systems, Inc., NY, USA) for holding the trunk. This type was assembled and tested with the aim of lowering the pressure and pain caused by the vertical slinging force around the hip and thigh. The supporting method at ischium, as used in the prosthetic socket for trans-femur amputees, is used in the design. A two-piece (front and rear) plastic shell was made to brace a thigh and to support the body weight at the ischium. The shells (left and right, front and rear) were connected to the vest with a non-elastic belt. This design reduced the feeling of oppression, it had a drawback of restricting the movement of the hip joint with the vest-to-shell attachment belts. The fault may have been solved if the belt alignment was appropriate, though there were other issues to be solved with the design.

The advantage of the ischium supporting method, improved version of Type I supporting vest, as shown in Fig 5, was discussed. A wooden bar covered by a foam rubber sheet with a curved surface to fit to the ischia was installed on top of the soft tube. See Fig.5 top left and right for its alignment. The pressure applied on the crouch is measured with an air package type contact surface pressure sensor (AMI techno Co. Ltd, Japan), with and without the bar. It was found that the bar holds up to approximately 60 % of the supporting force applied around the crouch area [10].

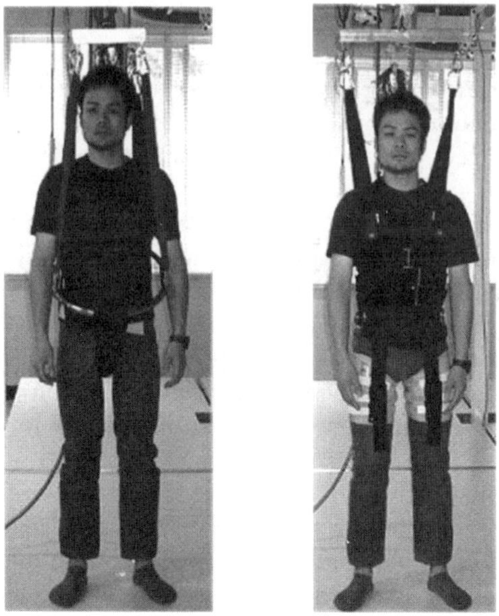

(a)Type I (b)Type II

Fig. 4. Supporting vest Type I (left) and Type II (right).

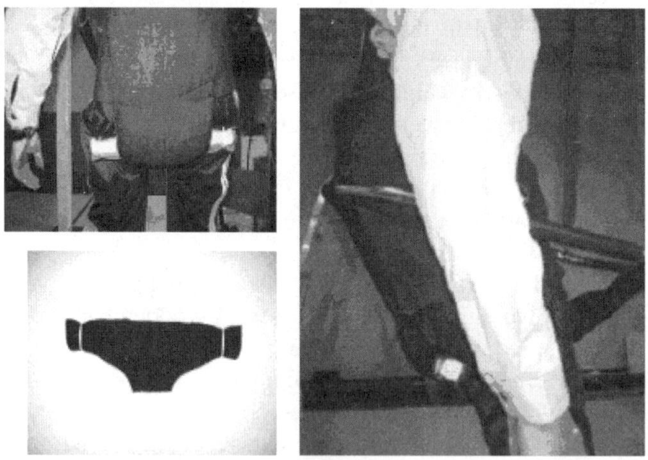

Fig. 5. Modified version of Supporting vest Type I, rear view (top left) and side view (right). The wooden bar covered by a foam rubber sheet with a curved surface to fit to the ischia. (bottom left)

3.4 Force Plate

The surface of a force plate is 2400*1400 mm^2, and six plates are arranged in 2 rows of 3 plates to consist a training area. The plate consists of an aluminum honey comb inner layer and carbon fiber outer wrapper. This structure enables the plate to be light and stiff. The weight of each plate is 57.2 kg. The force sensor is arranged in the four corners of each force plate. This light structure also provides sufficient performance with a moderately sensitive force sensor.

3.5 Reaction Force Measurement

First, all force plate sensors are initialized at the system start-up. After this process, the sensors are capable of measuring and computing the load on the force plates based on the calibration data. The output signals from the force plate sensors are amplified and converted to digital signals at the amplifier module for each of the 6 force plates. Then the signal is forwarded with a time-sharing process through a single line to the main control unit. The main control unit calculates the sling force from the ground reaction force data measured at the force plates. Then, the controller transmits the calculated data to the sling system component. A H8S microprocessor system (Renesas Technology Corp., Japan) was used for the CPU of the main control unit.

We use Spread Spectrum Wireless Data Communications for communication between the main control unit and sling system component. This wireless system can be used without hazard for medical appliances since the power output is 45mW, this is 0.06 of that of a cellular phone. Thus, this wireless system reduces the restrictions and issues of moving the sling system component without increasing the risk. We believe that the wireless control signal transmission is a necessity for rehabilitation mechatronic systems. This is especially true for devices that lift and carry subjects.

3.6 Control

Figure 6 shows the block diagram of the sling control system. The aim is to maintain the total vertical ground reaction force equivalent to a preset target load. The motor torque is computed from the error of the ground reaction force and preset load. Threshold is set around the target load to work as a dead zone block and prevent unstable oscillation of the motor caused by minimal errors. A torque signal is computed by adding the difference between the target and present load to the offset value. That is, the difference between the subject's weight and the preset load. This signal is sent to the sling system component used to support the patient. By utilizing this control algorithm, the body of the patient is lifted when the weight on his/her feet pushes on the plate. It is lowered when leaning or hanging on to the device. This produces an effect similart to a buoyancy in supporting the body weight.

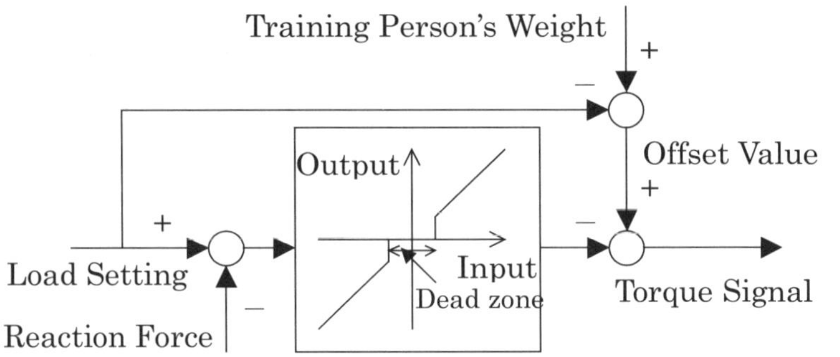

Fig. 6. The block diagram of sling force control.

4 Field Tests -Experimental Procedure and Results-

4.1 Pilot Testing

After some fundametal testing with unimpaired young subjects, the performance of the control system was tested with a healthy senior subject. The subject of this experiment was a female in her early seventies with a natural gait. Her weight was 461 N, and the support ratio is set to 35 %, the walking speed was set to 9.6 m/min. The slinging control was first shut off while the subject walked on the force plate. Then, the sling control was activated and the gait was measured with each of the two supporting vests. As seen in Fig.7, the results with sling control provide a support that can maintain the load equivalent to the target load, 300N, throughout the period, while the result of the gait without the control has an impulsive force at heel contact. Also, the supporting vest Type I shows a slightly better performance than Type II in the sense of minimizing variation. We assume that the result of Type II is due to the restricted leg movements that reduced the use of knee or hip joint for shock absorption.

The proposed control system demonstrated the capability of maintaining the supporting force near the target load of within 100 N error span in the experiments. The system has the expected control specification. The system needs improvement in order to be able to add adjustable parameters to set suitable control for the supporting vests.

The goal of the control strategy is to maintain a constant ground reaction force in the subject's gait. Therefore when the subject adds force to the feet, the sling controller increases the slinging force to lift the subject's body. Therefore, the controller reacts to assist the subject's vertical movement. In the experiment, we confirmed the controller that works by observing subject's body being slightly lifted when the toe was off the ground. Conversely, when the subject reduces the force on the feet, the controller releases the subject's body. As a result, the subject must always stand on his/her feet. The gain and maximum movable range of the sling force control system is limited for safety.

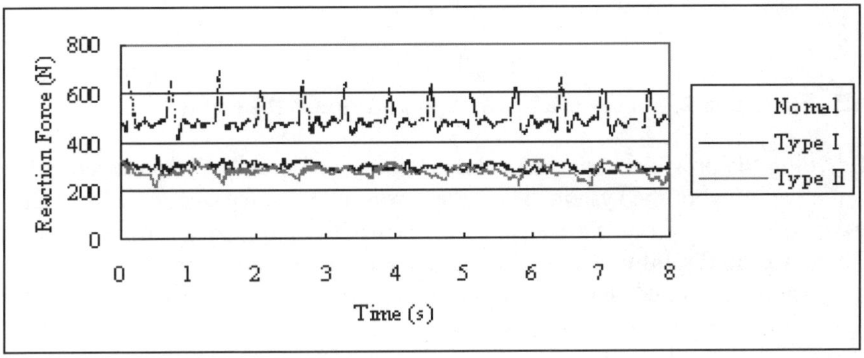

Fig. 7. The results of ground reaction force in the pilot experiment. The subject was a female adult in her early seventies with a natural gait. The results show that the sling control is capable of maintaining the requested support force and it can minimize the impulsive force at heel contact.

4.2 Field Test 1 –Sporadic Training on Multiple Subjects

The system was tested on unimpaired and impaired subjects with abnormal gait. Feedback was collected on the usability of the system. This includes factors such as the comfort of the vest. Five subjects were unimpaired, and seven subjects had feeble lower limb. The 5 impaired were in their 70's, four female and one male, and two, both male, were in their 50's. All of the impaired were capable of taking short walks on their own with a cane. Based on the level of disability and subject's condition, the supporting vest, load, and training period were predetermined. The subjects answered the questions on this questionnaire twice before and after the training.

Various experiments highlighted the following positive results:

- The system has no serious defects when used for gait training by those with feeble lower limbs. Adjustment of the load on the feet was accurately controlled by the system.
- The Type II vest is nearly painless even when the lifting force on the body is large. One minor drawback is the restriction of lower limb movement caused by the strap on the thigh.

- The characteristics of the subjects' gait patterns were quantifiable by following the graphical representation of the force plate sensor data. The patterns clearly differed and were based on the subjects' disabilities and their walking patterns. Almost all subjects remain stable while walked with the Type I vest.

The above data and comments provided useful feedback and was used to make minor modifications to the supporting vest and the experimental protocols.

4.3 Field Test 2 -Successive Training on a Impaired Person

Based on the previous experimental data, successive training was carried out to observe the effect of the system. The patient was a 25 year-of-age male, weighing 490 N, who suffered from partial paralysis on his left side caused by a brain tumor. There was no disability in the upper limbs. He had surgery in the past for his condition. He used a wheelchair for transportation and had had no gait training or walking experience apart from five years ago. This patient had enough muscular power to stand and to move both feet forward at the hip of the start of this testing. He could extend both knees and other joints fully, but did not have full control of the lower limbs because of the nervous disorder. Hence, the trainee could maintain a standing position for a short time but had difficulty in balancing during gait.

The subject trained 3 times a week for 10 days. In the beginning, two 5-minute training sessions were made with a 10-minute break in between. The preset load was set to 150 N, which was the maximum load that allowed the patient to walk naturally. Walking speed was set to 7.2 m/min so that the patient could step while confirming his position visually. The distance of the gait was approximately 36 m/test.

To evaluate the effects of the gait training device, CT, bone density, and lung capacity examinations, blood tests and patient feedback were taken for comparison before and after the training. The training period, preset load, and gait speed were increased when the subject requested. Verbal feedback was noted after each day of training.

System settings during the last training session were, load 200 N, gait speed 9.6 m/min and a training period of 10 minutes.

A type II vest was initially selected for use because it had wider contact area to reduce the body surface pressure. It was assumed that the Type I supporting vest would cause oppression on the crotch because of the high slinging force this patient needed. However, since the subject has to keep a catheter attached to his thigh, the shell on the thigh supporting vest Type II could not be used. Thus, the modified version of supporting vest Type I, in Fig.5, was used. Though this subject did not have a delicate sensation in the lower extremity and the modified version of the support vest Type I was the best choice for him.

Table 1 shows the results of the blood, biochemical, lung capacity, and bone density tests before and after the training period. The improvements in respiratory function and bone density need further research to determine their relation to the training. Similar results were reported by our medical director when training chronic spinal-cord-injury victims in the past. For this reason, we assume that an increase in these values reveals a positive tendency that can be used to monitor the effects of the training. Training was completed in a short period, and no signs of anemia, hemolysis, liver dysfunction, or kidney dysfunction were reported. The abnormal total bilirubin index was not at a level to be questionable. Also the patient did not report postural hypotension during training.

Table 1. Medical test results before and after training.

Tests		Before training	After Training
Blood Test		Normal	Normal
Biochemical Test		Normal	Abnormal total bilirubin Index
Respiratory function	Lung capacity	2820ml	3170ml
	1 second forced expiratory volume	2600ml	2780ml
Bone density		1485m/s	1500m/s

The trajectories of the point of the ground reaction force in a horizontal plane for the first, fourth, and tenth training days are shown in Fig.8~10. The diagrams are computed from the data collected from the middle plate of the three plates on one side of the row. This was selected because the gait trajectory is in a straight-line path. During the first training session, an undescended trajectory was observed when the weight shifted from the right foot to the left. In contrast, this tendency weakened at the forth and tenth training trajectories. This matches the awkward character in the early training. The subject's steps showed signs of adapting as the training continued. For example, wavering of the left ankle joint disappeared. The subject's comments were as follows:

- Greater satisfaction then using parallel bars, since our system provides a stronger sense of walking on one's own feet.
- Increased ease in getting in and out of the wheelchair because of the improvement in the proprioception of balance between body and feet.
- It was easy to control the training exertion because of easy setting of the computer parameters.

To compare the effects of our dynamic support to a static support, a trial without the sling control was performed by the same subject. As for the result, the patient felt extremely fatigued from the second lap, and complained that the training was difficult to continue for the same amount of time as with the dynamic support training.

Only one subject was available for field test 2 and the test for display usage. Therefore, a general conclusion can not be drawn from these results. It is important to understand that drawing a general conclusion with limited information can only result in an ill-defined answer that will not be suitable for patients with particular impairments. A step by step correspondence to each subject is the best way of providing a reliable general solution.

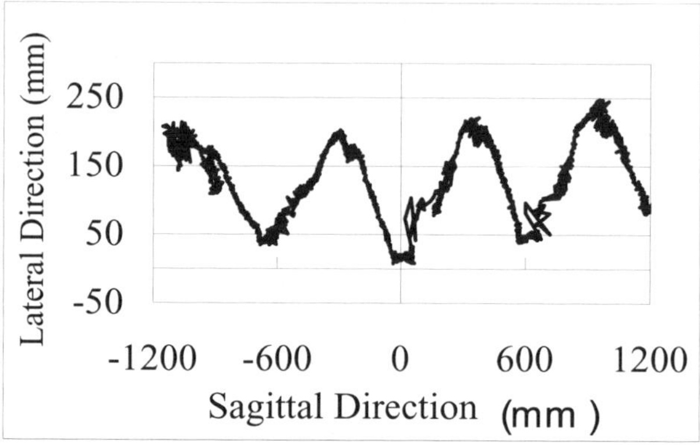

Fig. 8. The point of the reaction force in successive training on a impaired person. The first gait training day.

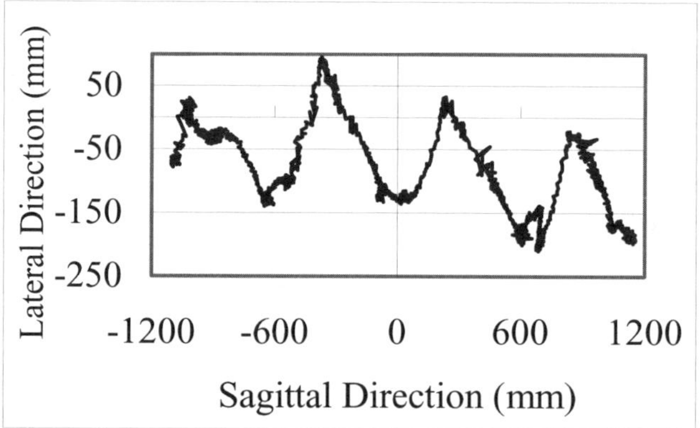

Fig. 9. The point of the reaction force in successive training on a impaired person. The fourth training day.

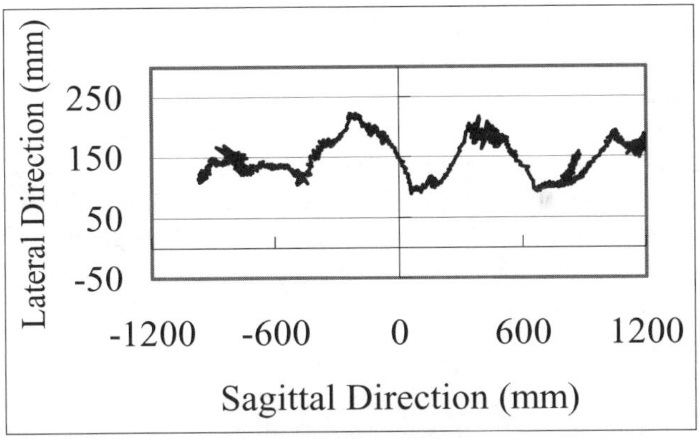

Fig. 10. The point of the reaction force in successive training on a impaired person. The tenth training day.

5 Walking Posture Assessments on Gait Training System

It was shown in the previous section that the effects of using our gait training system for impaired and elderly persons with lower physical ability was based on their comments and the recorded ground reaction force. In this section, walking posture of our gait training system is described by means of the experimental analysis comparing impaired and unimpaired subjects. First, the improvement of walking posture using an online camera-display system for impaired person is described. Secondly, the difference in the walking posture between natural walking and walking with the support of our gait training system is described.

5.1 The Effect using Display to subject with paralysis on Walking Posture

The same subject in the field test 2 was used for this testing. The protocol for the test was based on the field test 2. This testing followed the earlier test. Hence, the condition is similar to or more advanced than that of the last test. The analysis is done by computing the body posture from video data recorded in the training. The software used for computation is a three-dimensional video analysis system, Frame DIAS II (DKH Co., Ltd., Japan). This system consists of a 4 video camera recording system and processing software. We installed a XGA-LCD (SHARP Corp., Model:LL-T15G1, Japan) in front of the subject's head enabling him to monitor his steps while maintaining the view around the training area. A 0.3 Mega pixels CCD camera (KEYENCE Corp., Model:MC-1000, Japan), is installed at the bottom of the display facing the subject's feet. The camera captures the movement of his foot steps which he is able to watch while still looking ahead.

Stick pictures of the impaired person's posture in training are shown in Fig.11 and 12. These pictures were made from video data recorded when the patient was walking in a straight part of the training trajectory. Figure 11 and 12 are for the condition without a display. The posture in Fig.11 is poor due to the head leaning forwards. The subject is looking down and watching his steps to connect the sense of heel contact and foot position with his vision. The stick picture in Fig.12 is in a straight head-body alignment and is better than Fig.11. The subject's walking posture is maintained in a good condition as he is by looking forward.

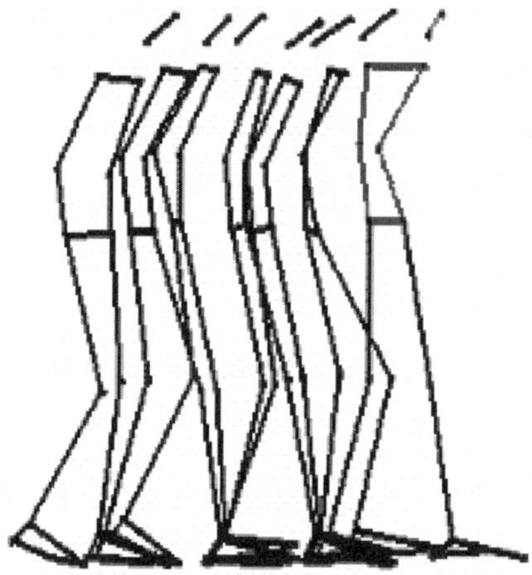

Fig.11. Stick picture of walking posture: walking while looking down

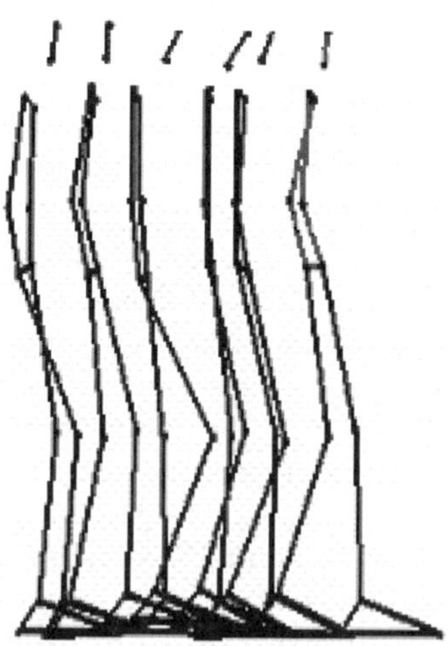

Fig.12. Stick picture of walking posture: Walking while looking ahead

Figure 13 and 14 show the difference of Center of the Pressure of the reaction force (COP) of the walk described above. Figure 13 is the COP while looking down. This trajectory is relatively stable. Figure 14 shows the COP when the patient is looking ahead. The COP is unstable and his body wobbles on, in other words loses control temporally. The subject commented that when looking forward he felt uneasy since he did lacked the feedback from his lower extremities.

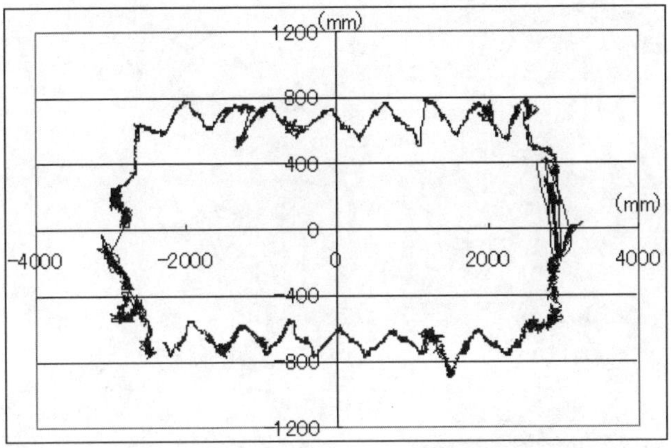

Fig.13. COP trajectory of training: walking while looking down

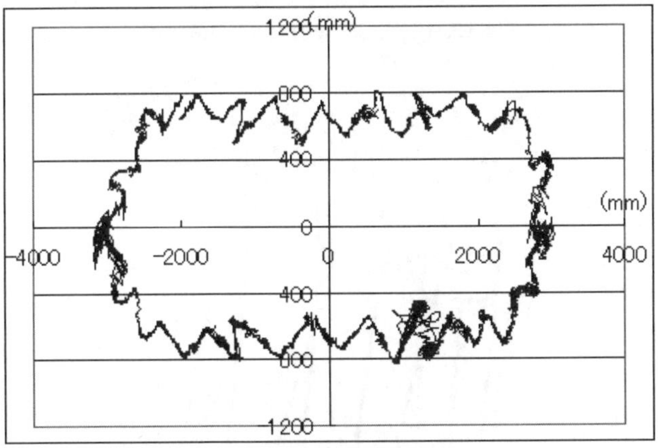

Fig.14. COP trajectory of training: walking while looking ahead

The subject's walking posture is satisfactory while looking ahead but the COP stability is better when looking down. The subject cannot sense the heel contact and the foot position because of paralysis. Therefore, he has to depend on visual feedback to stabily control his foot location for balance. If he looks down for stability his spine bends and his posture becomes inappropriate. In human walking, an upright posture is important. To continue the training with a poor posture can be harmful. A solution was therefore required to have good posture with the astable COP.

The testing arrangement is shown in Fig.15. The effect of using a stick is shown in Fig.16. The subject's posture is better than Fig.11 and close to Fig. 12.

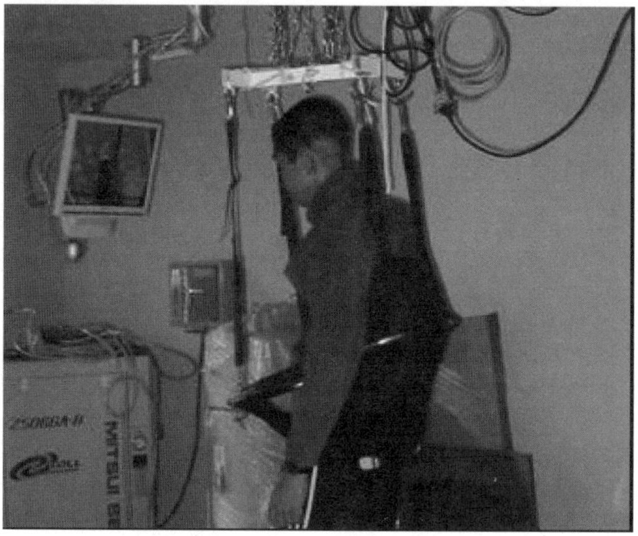

Fig.15. The LCD setting for the test.

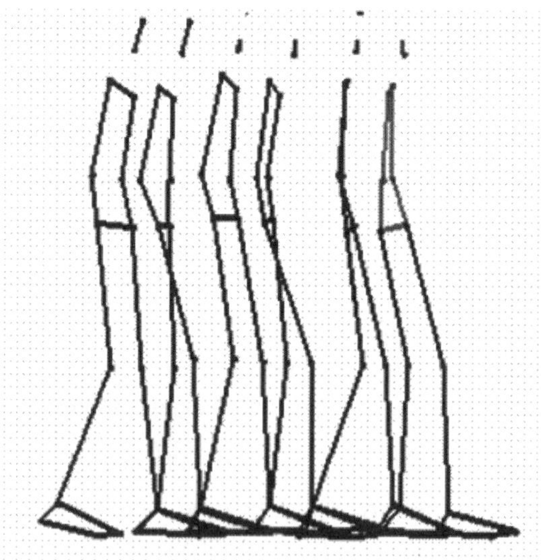

Fig.16. Walking posture on gait training system with LCD

Figure 17 shows the COP with the display. Fig.18 shows it without the display and the subject walking with the same step width as in Fig.17. Trajectory COP with the display is more stable than without the display. Table 2 is the angle of body or torso from vertical axis. This angle is calculated by Frame DIAS II. The angle of 'with display' is the best in this table. The angle of walking with display is also the smallest.

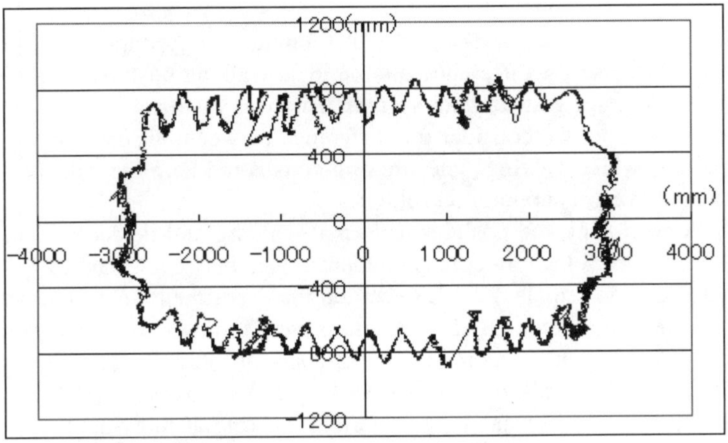

Fig.17. Trajectory of COP with the display

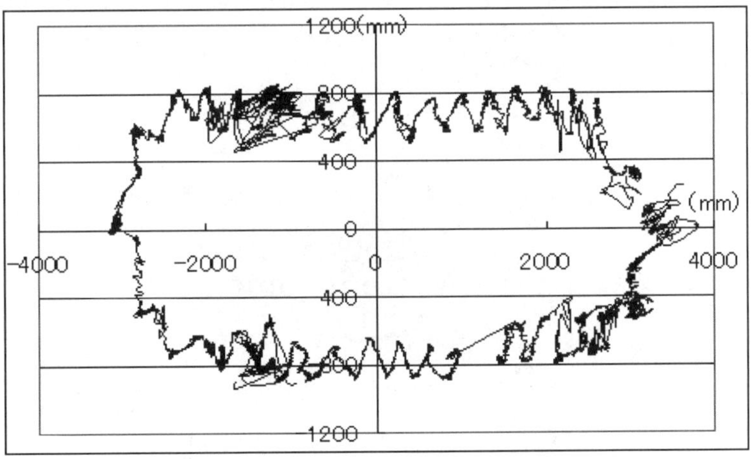

Fig.18. Trajectory of COP without the display (Step width is same as Fig.17)

Table 2. Angle of body from vertical axis (rad)

	Looking Down	Looking Ahead	With Display
Angle of body	0.64	0.27	0.16

5.2 The difference of Walking Posture: Normal vs Training System

A person's posture when walking in gait training is very important. However, the walking posture may be different from the ideal walking postures on a normal floor than when using our gait training system. This was confirmed in the previous section. In this section, we consider the difference between normal walking and using and apparatus while walking. The walking considered here are with the supporting vest and body weight support control.

In this experiment, the posture of normal walking and device walking is measured. Subjects are 5 healthy college students, ages between 22 and 24. Three were male and two were female. Each subject did the experiment once. The walking posture is measured by Frame DIAS II. Markers are fixed to parts of the subjects' body, and the 4 video cameras record the walk. There are three types of walking conditions, that is, device walking, normal walking at the constant speed guided by the gait training system (Normal-1), and normal walking at individual's normal speed (Normal-2). The speed of the device walking is slow compared to the normal speed, and set to correspond to the speed that the lower limb patients used.

We analyzed following data; the Center of Gravity (COG), the Range of Movement (ROM) of hip joint, ROM of the knee joint, maximum kicking height of the heel, angle of torso, and step length. Fig.19, 20, 21 and 22 show how these values were defined.

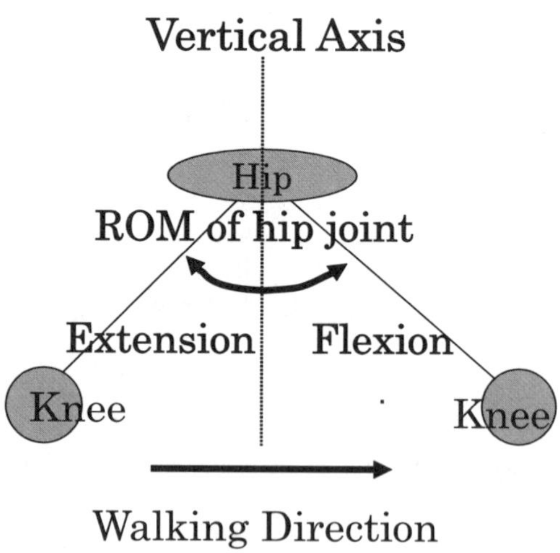

Fig.19 Definition of Range of Motion (ROM) of hip joint

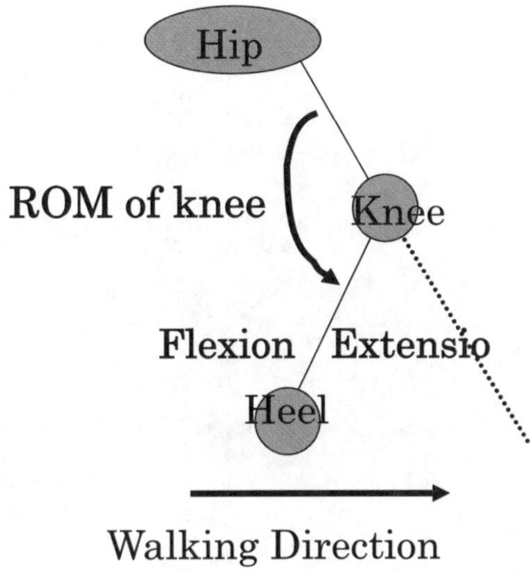

Fig.20 Definition of Range of Motion (ROM) of knee joint

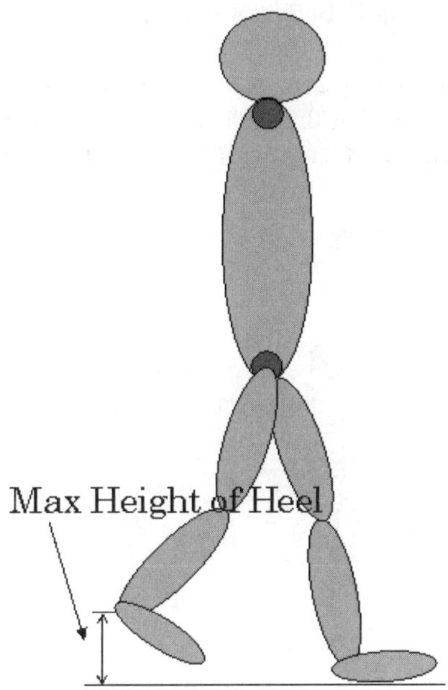

Fig.21 Definition of max height of heel

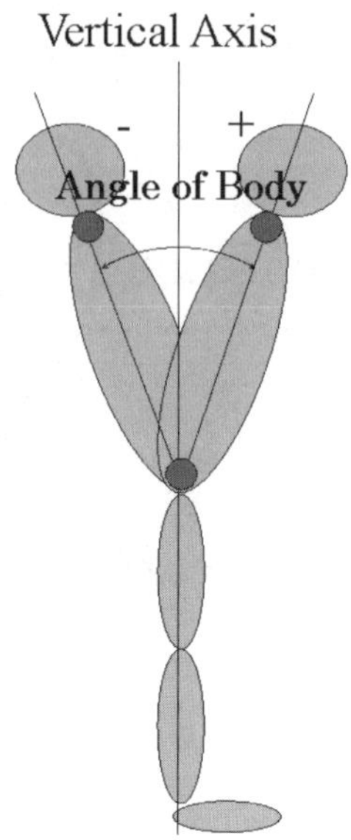

Fig.22 Definition of angle of torso

Figure.23, Fig.24, and Fig.25 show stick picture example of the 3 walking types. In device walking, we found that the torso was inclined and the knee joints did not become as straight as when compared with the normal walking.

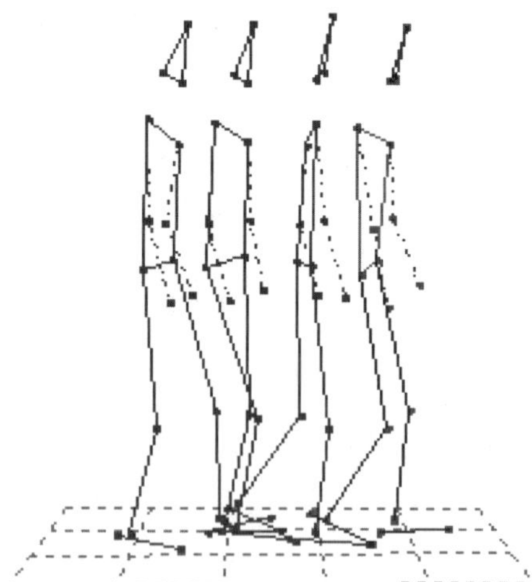

Fig.23 Stick pictures of device walking

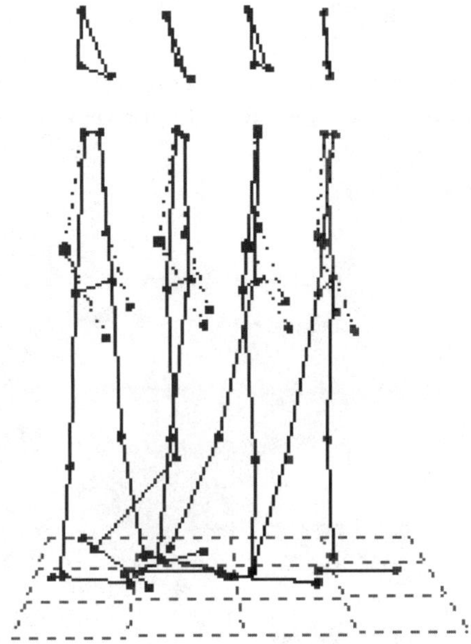

Fig.24 Stick pictures of Normal-1 (normal walking at a speed guided by the gait training system)

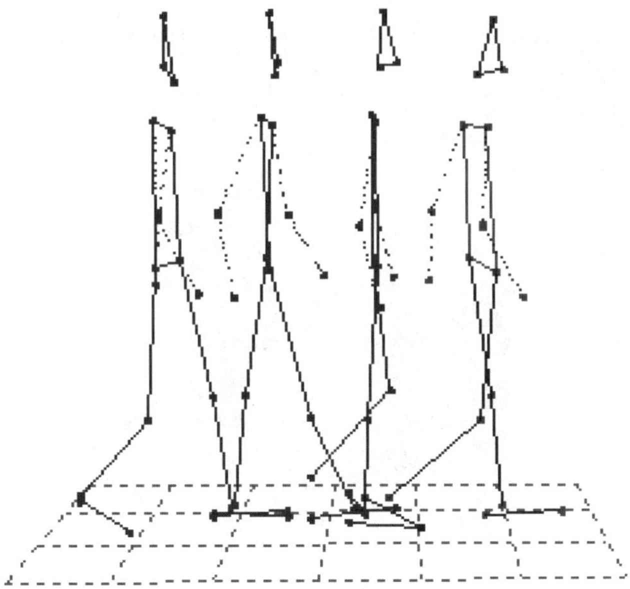

Fig.25 Stick pictures of Normal-2 (normal walking at normal speed)

Figure 26 shows the amplitude of the COG wave in lateral direction and Fig.27 shows the amplitude of the COG wave in vertical direction. The lateral direction amplitude in device walking is smaller than that of Normal-1 and is close to Normal-2. Vertical direction amplitude in device walking is smallest. The subject in device walking is assumed to be constrained by the support vest and slinging system.

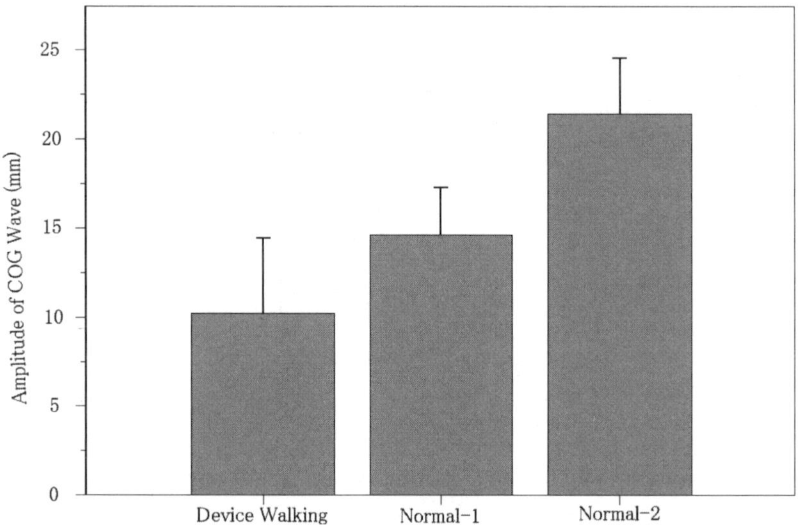

Fig.26 Average amplitude of the Center of Gravity (COG) wave in the lateral direction

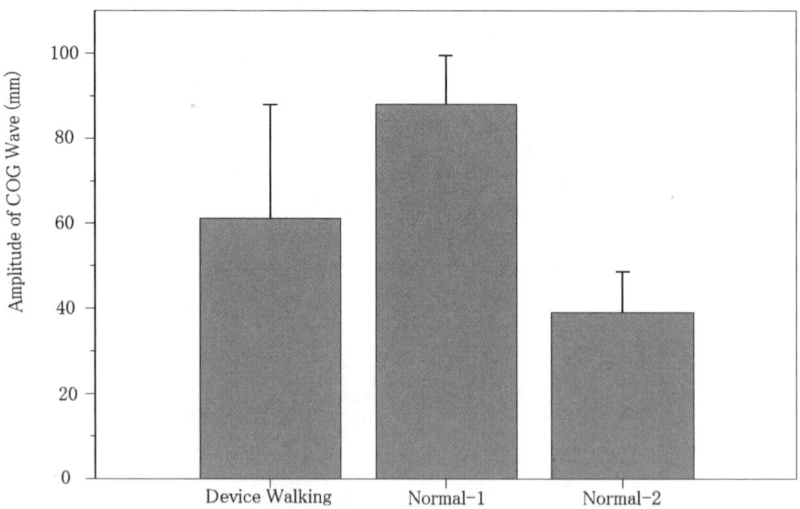

Fig.27 Average of the amplitude of Center of Gravity (COG) wave in a vertical direction

Figure 28 shows the ROM of the hip joint and Fig.29 shows the ROM of knee joint. Many subjects in device walking present smaller ROM than during normal walking conditions. For the hip joint, some of the subject's ROM in device walking is always positive.

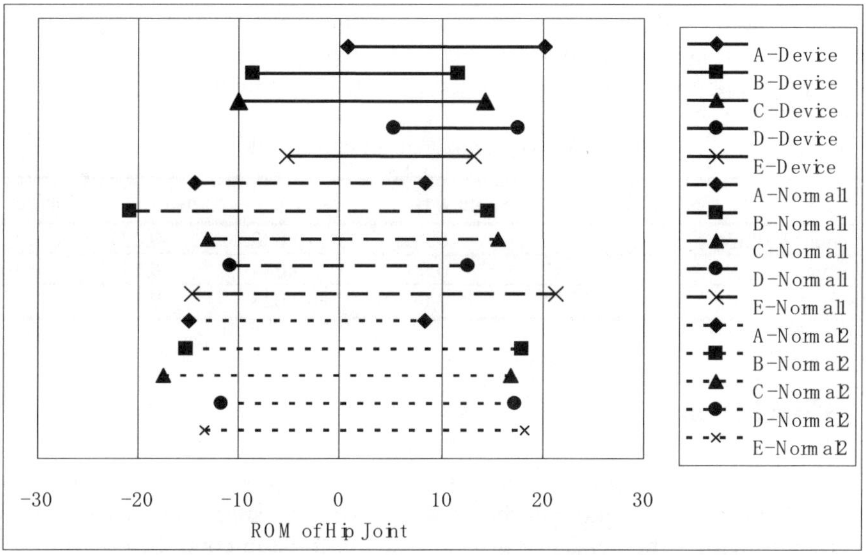

Fig.28 the Range of Motion (ROM) of the hip joint

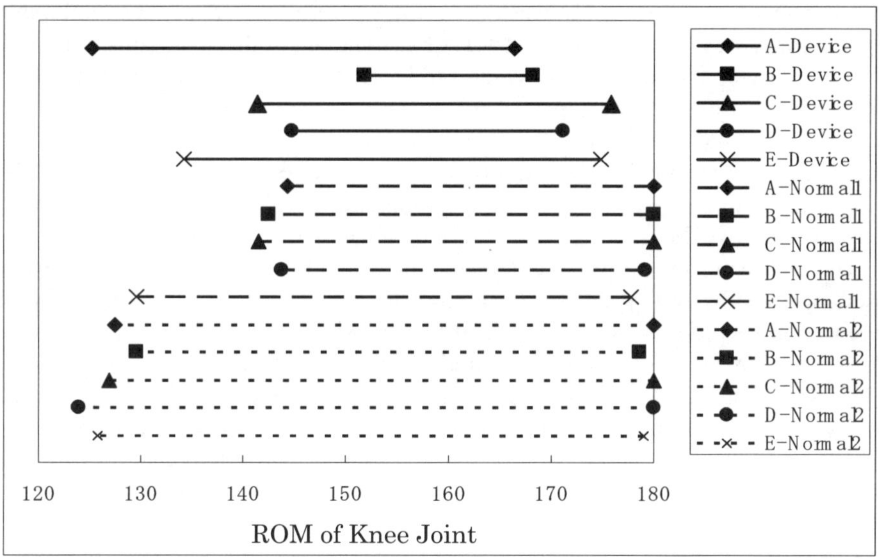

Fig.29 The Range of Motion (ROM) of the knee joint

Table.3 shows the torso angle of 3 walking types. The torso during device walking is inclined forward compared to normal walking conditions.

The maximum kicking height of the heel in device walking was smaller than under normal walking conditions, but this difference was small. The step length in device walking was equivalent or a little smaller when compared to Normal-1.

The quantitative difference of the device walking and normal walking is now described. Based on these quantitative findings we propose to improve the design of supporting vests and other modules of the gait training system.

Table 3. Average of angle of the torso (Rad)

	Subject A	Subject B	Subject C	Subject D	Subject E
Device Walking	0.072	0.264	-0.038	-0.037	-0.080
Normal 1	-0.017	0.007	-0.044	-0.148	-0.084
Normal 2	-0.005	0.000	-0.028	-0.126	-0.091

6 Conclusion

A unique gait-training device with a sling weight support system has been developed. The outstanding feature of this system is how the supporting tension holding the body to reduce the impact of ground reaction force in controlled. Performance tests showed that the control system is efficient in changing the ground reaction force around the preset load. The impact at the heel-contact and toe-off was reduced. Our control system produces the same sensation as independent walking by working in a way which is relaxing for the patient and at the same time it strengthens the muscles in his/her legs, which produces a vertical movement of the body. The floor reaction data from the system is useful in medical treatment, therapy, and other applications. Therefore, this innovative device, if mass-produced and marketed, could contribute to the rehabilitation of impaired people with feeble lower limbs. Interesting experimental results were obtained which show that setting a display can improve the walking posture of a paralized patient's gait.

The following results were obtained. The walking posture in impaired person was improved by setting display to monitor his step and the gait stability. The difference between device walking and normal walking was found. The person in the device walking was inclining compared with normal walking. The amplitude of COG wave, the ROM of the hip and knee joint and the average of kicking height of heel while in the device was smaller than that under normal walking conditions.

The findings of this research show that a computer controlled rehabilitation training systems is necessary to dramatically enhance rehabilitation techniques and it is better than conventional tools and training methods. Without such techniques, these systems are not practical with the system's cost and size. In further research work, we consider the following two functions to be indispensable features. The first is the fusion of the training function and the assessment function. Since our device has the force plate system for measuring the ground reaction force in a gait, we will explore combining an intelligent system which can automatically estimate the suitable slinging force from the force plate data and assess the efficiency of the locomotor therapy. Another feature is to enhance the subject's perception of his walking posture.

For practical implementation of these systems, the control and measurement performance needs improvement. The basic data gained in these test studies should be applied to improve the control algorithm, and the processing of the signal and test data. The modification of the control system and the effect on a human body is a challenging topic for further control engineering research.

It is necessary to improve the supporting vest and harnessing technique. The non-normal walking posture can be assumed to be produced to some extent as a by-effect of the vest's function and shape. Further investigations and modifications must be made as a result of further quantitative data to meet various subject body shapes and conditions.

Collaboration with the impaired and senior citizens is essential for research and experiments. Safety and reaction capacity constraints should never be underestimated in environment testing. Pilot testing on unimpaired subjects to gain reliable data for safety must be considered for each research topic and modification before proceeding to field testing with the impaired and elderly people.

Acknowledgement:

This work has been supported by a research project entitled “Rehabilitation System for Upper Limb and Lower Limb” through 1999-2004, a 5-year project founded by NEDO, Japan.

References

1. Kawamura, K., Ide, E., Hayashi, H., Ono, H. and Honda, T., Automatic suspension device for gait training, Prosthetics and Orthotics International, 1993; 17: 120-125.
2. http://www.fa-tec.co.jp/products/flora.htm (in Japanese)
3. Peshkin, M., Brown, DA, Santos-Munne, JJ, Makhlin, A, Lewis, E, Colgate, EC, Patton, J, Schwandt, D: KineAssist: A robotic overground gait and balance training device, International Conference on Rehabilitation Robotics, Proceedings CD-ROM, 2005, Paper WeD01.2.
4. Lee, C., Seo, K., Oh, C. and Lee, J., Newly Designed Rehabilitation Robot System for Walking-Aid with Pneumatic Actuator. International Journal of HWRS 2003; 4(1):42-46.
5. Gazzani, F., Bernardi, M., Macaluso, A., Coratella, D., Ditunno Jr, JF., Castellano, V., Torre, M., Macellari, V., Marchetti, M.: Ambulation training of neurological patients on the treadmill with a new Walking Assistance and Rehabilitation Device (WARD), Spinal Cord 37 1999: 336-344.
6. Kai, Y., Inoue, Y., Matsuda, T., Kawazawa, N., Sugawara, K., Ishida, K. and Yamamoto, H., A Study of Control Methods of a Sensor-Controlled Walking Support Machine on the

Basis of Leg Muscular Tensions during a Patient's Falling,The 2nd JSME Symposium on Welfare Engineering, 2002: 155-158, (In Japanese).

7. Egawa, S., Nemoto, Y., Koseki, A., Ishii, T., Fujie, MG.: Gait Improvement by Power-Assisted Walking Support Device, Human Friendly Mechatronics (ICMA 2000) 2001: 117-122.
8. Jezernik, S., Clombo, G., Keller, T., Frueh, H., Morari, M., Robotic Orthosis Lokomat: A Rehabilitation and Research Tool, Neuromodulation, Vol.6, No. 2, 2003: 108-115.
9. Tokyo Denki University: A Study of feedback type gait training system, New Energy and Industrial Development Organization Entrusted R&D Report for FY 1996 (in Japanese).
10. Imado, K., Miura A., Ikeuchi H., Ohnishi K., Nagatoshi M., Miyagawa H., Development of a unweighting vest for gait-training machines, proceeding of JSME Mechanical Engineering Congress 2002 Japan(MECJ-02), 2000; Vol.1: 93-94, (In Japanese).
11. Ikeuchi, H., Arakane, S., Ohnishi1, K., Imado, K., Saito, Y. and Miyagawa, H.: The Development of Gait Training System for Computer-aided Rehabilitation, Computers Helping People with Special Needs, 8th International Conference, ICCHP 2002 Linz, Austria, July 2002 Proceedings, 2002: 228-235.
12. Arakane, S., Ikeuchi, H., Ohnishi, K., Imado, K., Miyagawa, H. and Saito, Y., The Development and field test of Gait Training System, Proceedings of 6th Japan-France & 4th Asia-Europe Mechatronics Congress, Hatoyama, 2003: 147-152.
13. Ikeuchi ,H., Ohnishi, K., Imado, K, Miyagawa, H., Kamifukumoto,F. S. Arakane, S .and Saito, Y.: The assessments by trainees and an examination about walking posture on Gait Training System, Proceeding of 2004 IEEE/RSJ International Conference on Intelligent Robots and Systems, Sendai, Japan,2004: 1662-1667.